Eat to Feed

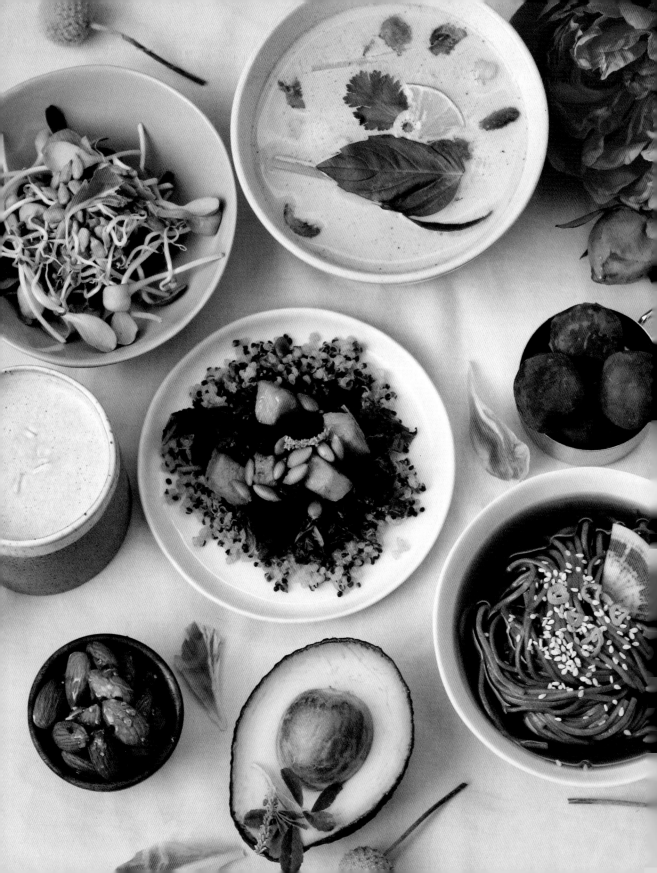

80 NOURISHING RECIPES FOR BREASTFEEDING MOMS

Eat to Feed

ELIZA LARSON AND **KRISTY KOHLER**

LIFE LONG

Copyright © 2019 by Kristy Kohler and Eliza Larson

Cover design by Endpaper Studio
Print book interior design by Endpaper Studio

Cover photograph by Eliza Larson

Cover copyright © 2019 Hachette Book Group, Inc.

Food photography by Eliza Larson. Breastfeeding photography on pages viii and 9 by Mary Salas.

Illustration credits: pages 35, 72, 122, 136, and 139 by Yuluck from the Noun Project; page 158 by Icons Producer from the Noun Project.

Da Capo Press
Hachette Book Group
1290 Avenue of the Americas
New York, NY 10104
www.dacapopress.com
@DaCapoPress

Printed in China

First Edition: July 2019

Published by Da Capo Press, an imprint of Perseus Books, LLC, a subsidiary of Hachette Book Group, Inc.

The Hachette Speakers Bureau provides a wide range of authors for speaking events. To find out more,
go to www.hachettespeakersbureau.com or call (866) 376-6591.

The publisher is not responsible for websites (or their content) that are not owned by the publisher.

Library of Congress Cataloging-in-Publication Data
Larson, Eliza, author.
Eat to feed: nourishing recipes for breastfeeding moms / Eliza Larson and Kristy Kohler.
First edition. New York, NY: Da Capo Lifelong Books, 2019.
Includes bibliographical references and index.
LCCN 2018051967
ISBN 9780738284873 (paperback)
ISBN 9780738284866 (ebook)
Breastfeeding. Mothers—Nutrition. Infants—Nutrition. Lactation—Nutritional aspects. Cookbooks.
LCC RJ216 .L338 2019 | DDC 649/.33—dc23
LC record available at https://lccn.loc.gov/2018051967

IM

10 9 8 7 6 5 4 3 2

To all mothers

CONTENTS

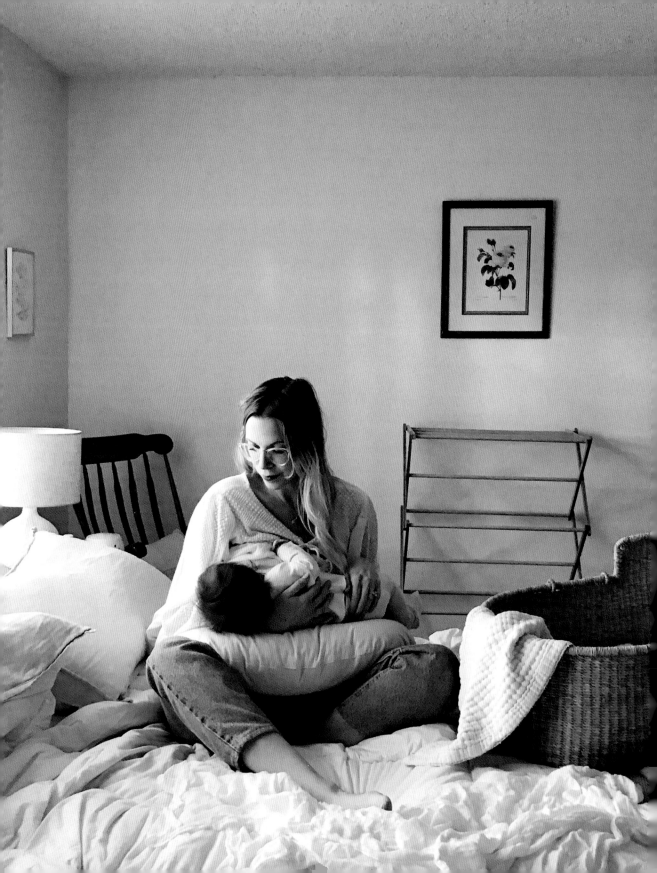

INTRODUCTION

Feeding is an act of love.

There are few things in life that compare to your baby falling asleep against your breast smiling, or looking right into your eyes while making sweet chortling noises. As a breastfeeding mom, you are sharing your body, your nutrients, and your food with your baby. But breastfeeding isn't easy—and that surprised both of us when we were new moms. (Nobody tells you breastfeeding will hurt!) When you're getting started breastfeeding, you need all the support you can get. We know this firsthand.

We met at a park while we were each pregnant with our second baby and quickly bonded over our choice of names. (Eliza's first son is named Oliver, and she was going to name her second boy Henry. Kristy's first son is named Henry, and her second son was going to be named Oliver. You know what they say about great minds!)

When our second babies were born, we both started nursing again. But Kristy was having a hard time producing enough milk, and Eliza had had trouble the first time around.

While we were dealing with nursing challenges, we had read extensively about ingredients called galactogogues: whole foods and herbs traditionally incorporated in a postpartum diet to help support a healthy milk supply. Many of these ingredients were unfamiliar to us at first. A few of them, such as brewer's yeast, were ones we hadn't cooked with at all.

After talking to lots of mom friends, we realized we were not alone in our confusion. Most of us turned to either taking supplements or steeping herbs in water to make bitter teas. Around this same time, we noticed a growing trend of lactation cookies in stores, but many of them weren't so tasty, or had lots of filler ingredients that aren't so good for you. That's where the inspiration for our lactation foods company, Oat Mama, was born.

Instead of choking down bitter teas or snacking on unhealthy cookies, we wanted to fill the postpartum period with foods that left us feeling cared for and energized. We decided to develop an incredibly tasty granola bar that was free of dairy, soy, and gluten; filled with galactogogues, such as brewer's yeast and ground flax; and packed with healthy fats from nuts, seeds, and coconut oil. The first Oat Mama bar was born, and the reaction from moms was overwhelming. From there we took our mission further. We updated traditional grassy lactation teas with our line of Oat Mama teas featuring punchy fruit flavors, such as Blueberry Pomegranate, so they could be enjoyed hot or iced. As breastfeeding moms ourselves, we continue to think about what real moms actually want to eat and drink and what products will bring more health and enjoyment to nursing.

We also deeply care about community. Since support is one of the top predictors of breastfeeding success, we knew we wanted to incorporate as much support into our brand as possible. With our very first message of "You Got This" on our original bars to our vibrant community of moms on our social media feeds and Facebook group, we wanted every mom to feel connected and encouraged through her unique breastfeeding journey. We created the hashtag #mothertogether in this spirit and also donate a portion of our sales to help deliver lifesaving donor breast milk to babies in the NICU. Since the beginning, we've also developed and shared lactation recipes on our Oat Mama blog. Here's what one mama said about our Coconut Panna Cotta: "Since most desserts are light on the fat and high on the sweetener, this is a great way to have a healthy dessert that feels like a treat but still has good nutrition in it. Panna Cotta beats Jell-O any day and is far more filling than the sugary, store-bought options with only a few minutes work." The incredible response and demand for these nourishing lactogenic recipes led us to creating *Eat to Feed*.

We wrote *Eat to Feed* not only to demystify galactogogues but also to celebrate their unique flavor profiles and nutritional content. As passionate food enthusiasts, our goal was to come up with innovative and extremely tasty ways of cooking with these ingredients. All of our recipes highlight specific galactogogues in easy-to-use, delicious preparations that were created with you in mind.

By no means do you need or require a "perfect" diet to successfully breastfeed—not at all. There is no pressure or expectation here. And note that if you are encountering breastfeeding issues, food alone cannot "fix" low supply. We strongly believe that there is *no* substitute for best breastfeeding practices (feeding on demand, correct latching, skin-to-skin contact), good counsel from a professional lactation consultant or La Leche League leader, or meeting with a local breastfeeding support group to get you and your baby off to the strongest start possible. With *Eat to Feed*, we want to offer you a chance to broaden your culinary horizons and mark this special—and fleeting—time in your life with the smell and tastes of dishes you'll always remember fondly as part of your journey as a new mother. Our hope is that you'll continue turning to these superfoods and the recipes in this book long after your little ones have weaned.

By keeping yourself well nourished, well hydrated, and well rested, you are better equipped to navigate the inevitable ups and downs of feeding your baby. Nourishing yourself, and making that a priority, is the greatest gift you can give your baby. And it's a good first step toward building a healthy family with a positive attitude about food. We hope these recipes delight you, comfort you, and remind you that you are not alone in this, and that every act of feeding yourself and your baby is one of pure love.

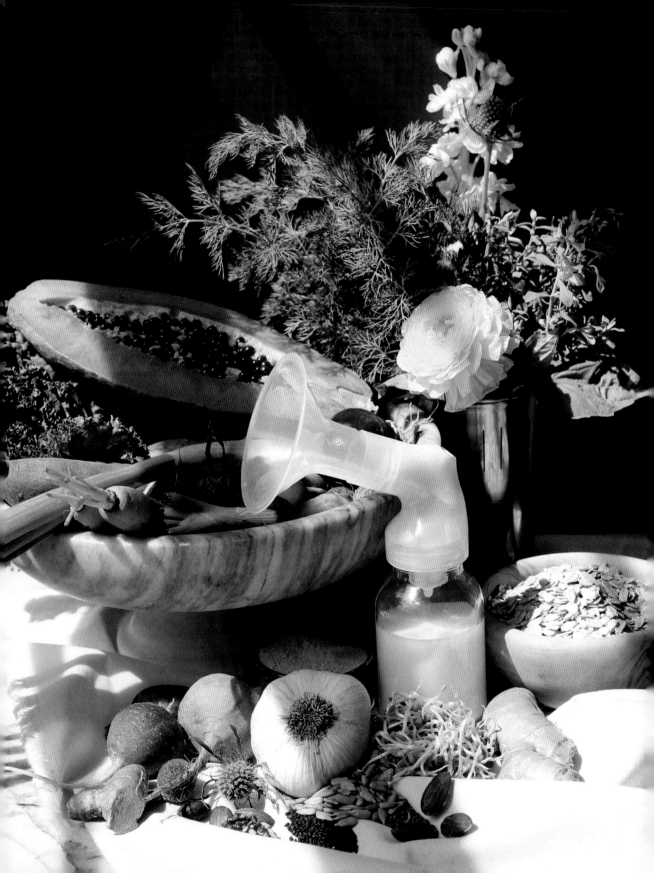

STOCKING YOUR PANTRY

Your Guide to Galactogogues and Other Key Ingredients for Breastfeeding

The recipes in this book feature amazing ingredients that can help to support a healthy body and a healthy milk supply while you are nursing your little one. Certain of these ingredients are galactogogues: foods and herbs that naturally boost milk production. Others are featured because they contain lots of powerful vitamins, minerals, and other compounds that may help you to keep up your health and energy when you're breastfeeding. Throughout the book, you'll see a drop icon that highlights the main galactogogues or milk-boosting ingredients in any given recipe.

Galactogogues are often taken in the form of supplements or teas. But they can also be made into delicious homemade foods and drinks—and that makes them not only more fun for you to eat, but to share with your family, too. (And don't worry, there's absolutely no harm in sharing any of these delicious ingredients and dishes with your kids or your partner. There's no "mystery estrogen" here—they're all healthful foods made from whole, honest ingredients that are good for just about anyone, but they offer breastfeeding moms a bonus!)

Before we go any further, we should acknowledge that scientists and researchers have studied various galactogogues, and their findings are inconclusive. As such, the lactogenic effects of these foods are generally not scientifically proven—more studies would be needed to determine how they work and just how effective they are. Most of what we know about galactogogues is based on anecdotal evidence shared among mothers, and passed down through generations of kitchen wisdom. We're building on what we found in our own research, plus the wisdom we've gained talking to other wonderful mamas in our real-life and online communities. Over the years, we've used ourselves as guinea pigs, and gotten feedback from others, so we know what's worked for many of us—and now, we share it in the hopes that it can help you, too.

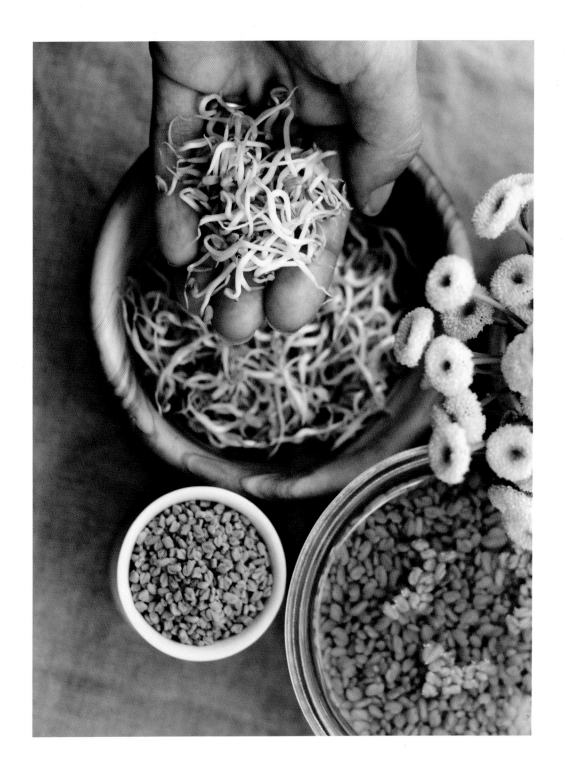

GRAINS AND FLOURS: organic oats, barley, buckwheat, black rice, brown rice, quinoa, millet, bulgur

Probably the most widespread advice mothers receive, besides maybe to drink a beer, is to eat lots of oatmeal. There are many reasons that the mighty oat has become the queen of lactogenic foods. It contains beta-glucans, fiber, iron, and protein, and research suggests it has a calming effect on the nervous system. When choosing oats, we always recommend organic. The other grains in this category are mighty as well, and most of them can be incorporated in the same diverse ways that oats can. Try them raw, toasted, soaked, cooked, made into milk, ground into flour, baked into cookies, and so on. The possibilities are exciting and endless. You're sure to find preparations that speak to your palate.

SPICES, HERBS, AND YEASTS: anise, basil, fennel seed, fenugreek, turmeric, ginger, dill, cumin, garlic, brewer's yeast, nutritional yeast

Spices are literally the spice of life! Time-honored and widely-recognized galactogogues, such as fenugreek, fennel, ginger, and anise, are commonly found in many lactation teas and supplements on the market. Others, such as turmeric, help to rid the body of inflammation. In a study published in *Pediatrics*, babies were shown to nurse longer after a mom has eaten garlic. Cumin seeds are packed with iron that may help stave off postpartum anemia, which can lead to low milk supply. Dill and basil are rich in vitamin K and antioxidants. Brewer's yeast and nutritional yeast are packed with B-complex vitamins, amino acids, and minerals. These can specifically aid in fighting off postpartum depression, boosting immunity, and giving you beautiful hair, nails, and skin. You can find many of these herbs in their fresh forms or widely available in a dried powder. Yeasts are generally found either in the supplement aisle or bulk bins of grocery stores or online.

NUTS AND SEEDS: almonds, cashews, chia seeds, sunflower seeds, flaxseeds, black sesame seeds, white sesame seeds, hemp seeds, poppy seeds, pumpkin seeds

When we've polled breastfeeding moms about their healthy snacking habits, the number one answer is usually nuts and seeds. Nuts and seeds are quick, filling foods packed with protein and healthy fats (and you can generally eat them with one hand, no small consideration for someone with a babe in the other arm!). These nuts and seeds are lactogenic superstars providing fiber, delivering omega-3s, and calcium without excess sugar. And essential omega-3 fatty acids can be passed on through breast milk to your baby. While nuts and seeds are an ideal snack on their own, have fun experimenting in your kitchen with different nut and seed butters, oils, and milks as well. Most nut and seed butters can be created by simply placing the raw or toasted ingredients in a high-powered blender and pulsing until the oils have released and the mixture becomes creamy.

FRUITS AND VEGETABLES: apricots, figs, dates, coconut, papayas, asparagus, avocados, kale, spinach, moringa, beets, carrots, fennel, sweet potatoes, pumpkin, squash, dried seaweed

Leafy greens, such as kale and spinach, are an essential part of a healthy postpartum diet, or any diet, for that matter. But leafy greens are especially important for new moms to fight off post-pregnancy anemia and for their phytoestrogen content. Dried fruits are a great source of energy and calcium. Orange root vegetables are full of vitamin A and beta-carotene, and concentrated amounts can be found in a mom's first colostrum, otherwise known as "liquid gold." Dried seaweed, and broth made from it, is a beloved postpartum healing food in many Asian cultures due to seaweed's high iodine content and protective antioxidants.

EGGS AND DAIRY: eggs, full-fat Greek yogurt

Eggs are rich in choline, a substance that is naturally occurring in breast milk and is critical for early development. Eggs and yogurt are high-protein foods. Yogurt has the additional benefit of contributing to a healthy gut flora for mom and baby while providing a boost of calcium.

BEANS AND PULSES: chickpeas, lentils, peas

Beans, lentils, and peas are not only filling, but eaten alongside whole grains or nuts and seeds, they make a complete protein—and if you're eating a mainly plant-based diet, that is essential. Together they help deliver all essential amino acids. They deliver iron and help stabilize blood sugar levels. Not to mention, beans, lentils, and peas make mouthwatering salads, dips, spreads, taco fillings, and soups. You can also dehydrate them to make crunchy snacks.

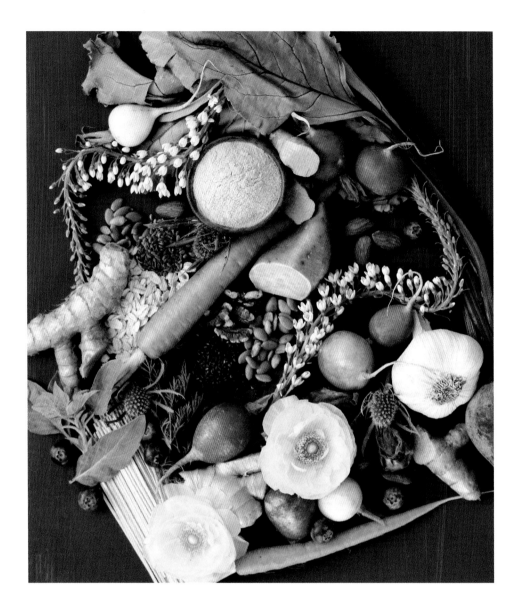

FATS AND SWEETENERS: extra-virgin coconut oil, extra-virgin olive oil, sesame oil, sunflower oil, grass-fed butter, molasses, coconut sugar, dates

Healthy fats deliver so many benefits to new moms, from lowering the risk of postpartum depression to helping baby's brain development. Breastfeeding moms should not look for ways to cut out fats from their diet, but do choose

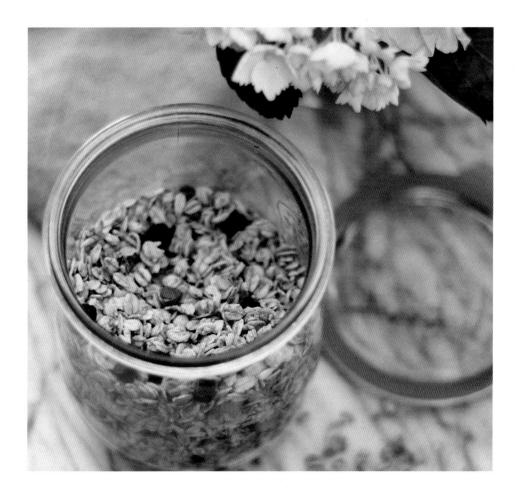

the good ones derived from nuts, seeds, coconut, and avocado. Treats are part of every balanced diet, but again, choosing sweets made from natural sweeteners or dried fruit offer some nutrients along with the calories.

NOTE: If you are having any problems with breastfeeding or low milk supply, food alone will not address any underlying issues. We strongly believe that there is *no* substitute for best breastfeeding practices (feeding on demand, correct latching, skin-to-skin contact), good counsel from a professional lactation consultant or La Leche League leader, or meeting with a local breastfeeding support group. This book is not intended as a replacement for professional lactation support.

BREASTFEEDING TIPS
from Lactation Consultants

We can't say it enough: breastfeeding is hard work. And though this isn't a breastfeeding guide—there are lots of good ones already out there!—we want to offer you some tips to get you started. With that in mind, we enlisted lactation consultants Crissi Blake and Nina Isaac to offer these helpful hints.

Breastmilk is the perfect food for babies, and is easily and quickly digested. Babies also have a tiny stomach, so, it is expected that they will need to feed more often than older kids and adults. Newborn babies seem to nurse all the time; this is normal! You may feel as though you are nursing constantly, and that is okay as long as your baby is growing well, having plenty of wet/dirty diapers, and meeting all developmental milestones. Typical breastfed babies feed at least every one to three hours.

Getting help and support early on will benefit the longevity of your nursing relationship. Look for a lactation professional or IBCLC (International Board Certified Lactation Consultant) in your community and give that person a call! Some women also find breastfeeding support groups very helpful. Look to see if there is one in your community.

TIPS:

• After delivery, hold your baby skin to skin as much as possible and ask for assistance latching when he or she is showing readiness cues.

• Breastfeed often, long, and on demand. This will ensure an abundant milk supply.

• Watch your baby's cues, instead of the clock, to ensure your child's satiation and determine when and how often to feed. This will not only help your baby get the milk he or she needs to grow and thrive, but it will also help your body *make* enough milk for your infant's needs.

• Make sure your baby is latched well and breastfeeding efficiently. This will help establish and maintain your milk supply.

- Offer both breasts with every feeding. This will ensure adequate stimulation of your breasts, which in turn ensures a good milk supply. As your baby gets older, both breasts may not be stimulated at every feeding. This is especially true as your little one becomes more efficient at breastfeeding.

- Make sure you are comfortable and relaxed when latching your baby. You may need to experiment with lots of different positions; find the one that works best for you both.

- When positioning your baby, hold him or her close to your body, tummy to tummy and nipple to nose, to ensure a deep and comfortable latch. If you experience discomfort, try leaning back slightly or change your position.

- There's no need to limit time at the breast. Let your baby nurse until he or she appears content, calm, and peaceful. Make sure to offer the second breast every time, especially in the early days and weeks of breastfeeding.

- Your pumping output is not indicative of your actual milk supply. Your baby is often more efficient than the pump. Many moms who don't respond well to the pump still do have an abundant milk supply. If your baby is growing well with adequate output, you have plenty of milk.

- Galactogogues (foods and herbs that help to increase milk supply; see page 1) can be used in addition to proper and efficient stimulation of your breasts, either by your baby and/or your pump, if you are struggling with milk supply.

- Eat when you're hungry and drink when you're thirsty. There are typically no specific foods you need to avoid while breastfeeding your baby.

- Be sure to take care of sore nipples. You can use your own breastmilk on your nipples in addition to a lubricating layer, such as coconut oil or your favorite nipple cream.

- Involve your partner in the breastfeeding relationship by asking for support with positioning, refilling your water, or bringing you a snack. Partners are also wonderful at changing diapers, bathing the baby when needed, and holding the child skin to skin after feeds.

Give yourself permission to take breastfeeding one day at a time. Celebrate all of the little successes and know you are not alone. And it's okay to ask for help when you need it.

Written by Crissi Blake RN, BSN, IBCLC, and Nina Isaac MS, CCC-SLP, IBCLC. Owners of Milk and Honey Specialized Breastfeeding and Postpartum Support Center, Tucson, AZ. www.milkandhoneytucson.com

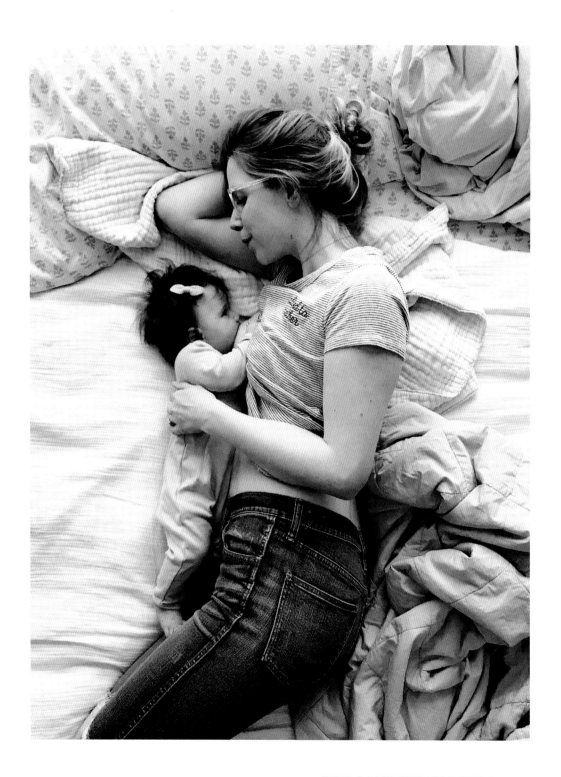

Breakfast

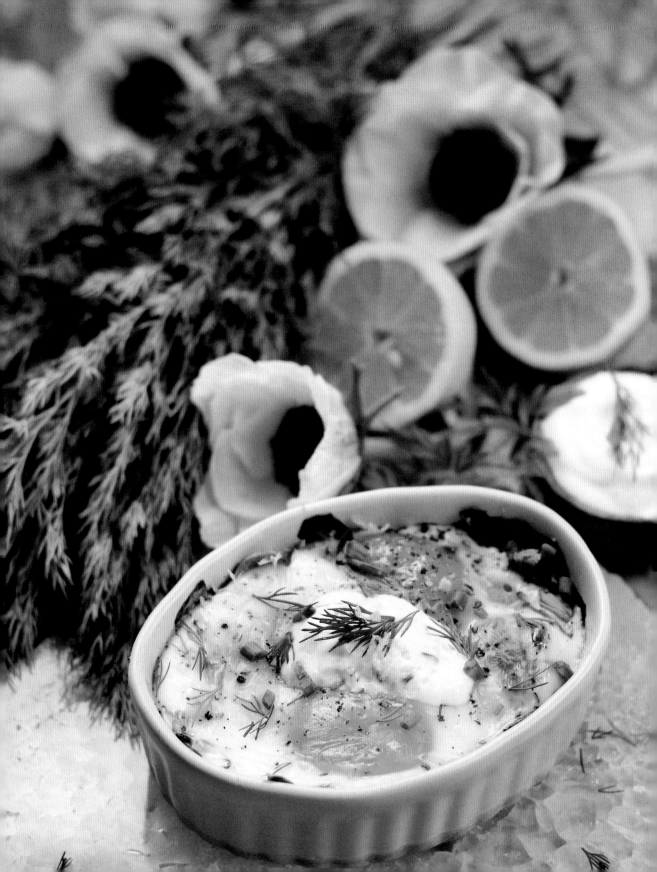

BAKED EGGS with YOGURT AND DILL

spinach, eggs, Greek yogurt, dill

While we love eggs over here, many classic egg dishes are loaded with cheese and grease and can leave you feeling sluggish. Here is a high-protein breakfast packed with healthy fats that won't weigh you down. Fresh dill, scallion, and lemon zest give these eggs a bright, cheerful disposition. Most baked egg recipes use only heavy cream. We added a dollop of Greek yogurt after baking for its healthy fat, protein, and probiotics. (We also put two eggs in each ramekin because, hey, breastfeeding hunger is real.) We like to sop up those yolks with a slice of toasty bread. Yum.

SERVES 4

Unsalted butter, for ramekins

2 cups lightly packed spinach

¼ cup heavy cream

Salt and freshly ground black pepper

8 large eggs

¼ cup full-fat Greek yogurt

2 tablespoons chopped fresh dill

¼ cup chopped scallion

2 teaspoons lemon zest

1. Preheat the oven to 350°F. Grease four 6-ounce ramekins lightly with butter.

2. Fill the bottom of each ramekin with ½ cup of the spinach and pour 1 tablespoon of the cream over the spinach in each ramekin. Season each with a grind of pepper and a pinch of salt.

3. Crack two eggs into each ramekin. Lightly season each again with a pinch of salt and a grind of pepper.

4. Place the ramekins on a cookie sheet in the middle rack of the oven. Bake for 18 to 20 minutes, or until the egg whites are set but the yolks are still runny.

5. Remove from the oven and top each ramekin with 1 tablespoon of Greek yogurt, 1½ teaspoons of dill, 1 tablespoon of scallion, and ½ teaspoon of lemon zest. Serve immediately.

CARROT PESTO EGG TOAST

carrot, basil, garlic, nutritional yeast

We fell hard for this carrot pesto. It has now become a staple in our fridges. It's so quick to put together, and can turn a ho-hum piece of toast into something that feels very fancy and sophisticated. Sometimes we are just not up to going out to eat with a nursing baby and all the gear it can require, but we'd still like to experience a restaurant-worthy meal at home. The bright orange pesto makes for such a pretty breakfast you'll feel as if you're splurging, and only you'll know how easy it was to make.

CARROT PESTO:

MAKES ABOUT ½ CUP PESTO

1 medium-size carrot, chopped

¼ cup packed fresh basil

3 garlic cloves

3 tablespoons pine nuts

3 tablespoons nutritional yeast

⅛ teaspoon salt

PER TOAST:

MAKES 1 SERVING

Olive oil

1 large egg

Salt and freshly ground black pepper

1 slice whole-grain or seeded bread

1 tablespoon carrot pesto

1. Prepare the carrot pesto: Place the carrot, basil, garlic, pine nuts, nutritional yeast, and salt in a food processor and blend for about 30 seconds, or until it forms a paste. Add more salt to taste.

2. To prepare each toast: Pour a light drizzle of olive oil into a skillet over medium-high heat and heat for 1 to 2 minutes.

3. Crack the egg into the hot oil and sprinkle a pinch each of salt and pepper on top. Cook the egg to your preferred taste, 1 to 2 minutes for a runny yolk, longer for a more cooked egg.

4. Meanwhile, toast the bread.

5. Slather a tablespoon of pesto over the toasted bread and top with the fried egg. Enjoy immediately.

6. Store the remainder of the pesto in an airtight container in the refrigerator for up to a week.

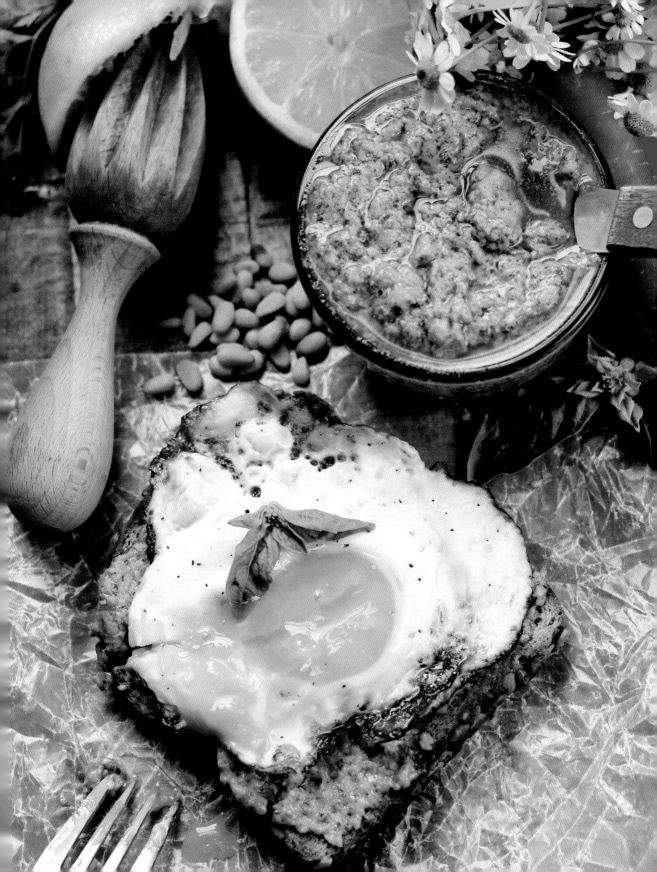

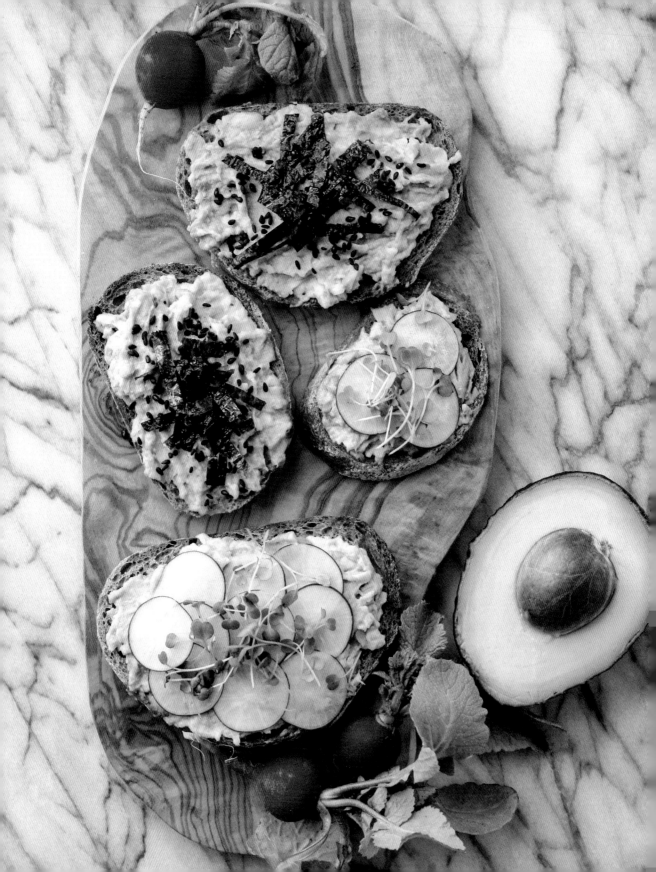

AVOCADO TOAST TWO WAYS

sesame, seaweed, nutritional yeast

Avocado toast has earned its place at breakfast tables across the country, and for good reason. Not only is it simple, beautiful, and tasty, but there are about a hundred and one ways to do avocado toast. Of course, we had to give you our versions. The first gets an extra boost of protein from edamame and sesame, and the other delivers B vitamins and iron from the nutritional yeast. Both are equally yummy, and can be easily shared with nearby babies and toddlers.

Sesame Avocado Toast

SERVES 1

½ avocado, pitted and peeled

1 tablespoon cooked, cooled, and shelled edamame

Pinch of salt

Drop of sesame oil (optional)

1 slice seeded or multigrain bread, toasted

½ teaspoon sesame seeds (we use a mixture of white and black)

2 sheets toasted seaweed snack, cut into matchsticks

Smash the avocado and edamame together with the salt and sesame oil, if using. Spread on top of the toast and sprinkle with the sesame seeds and seaweed. Enjoy immediately.

Buttery Avocado Toast

SERVES 1

½ avocado, pitted and peeled

½ teaspoon nutritional yeast

Pinch of salt

1 slice seeded or multigrain bread, toasted

1 radish, sliced thinly

Microgreens (optional)

Smash the avocado and nutritional yeast together with the salt. Spread on top of the toast. Top with the radish slices and microgreens, if using. Enjoy immediately.

OVERNIGHT BREAKFAST BULGUR

bulgur, almond milk

We've all been told we need to eat breakfast, and this is especially true for nursing moms. The only problem is finding time—and free hands—to whip up something that is healthy, satisfying, and easy. You may already know about overnight oats by now, but there are a few other quick-cooking grains that soften while you sleep (or breastfeed) and are ready first thing in the morning. If you haven't tried bulgur yet, you're going to love it. Its pleasant chew is reminiscent of steel-cut oats. The almond milk adds a slight creaminess without being overly heavy. Doll it up any way you like; we enjoy ours straight from the fridge with fresh berries and a splash of coconut milk. Also try it warmed up, topped with maple syrup, sliced almonds, and a sprinkle of cinnamon.

SERVES 1 TO 2

⅓ cup uncooked bulgur

⅓ cup almond milk

In a bowl or jar with a lid, combine the bulgur with the almond milk and ⅓ cup of water, cover, and place in the fridge for 6 to 8 hours or overnight. Serve cold or lightly heated as desired.

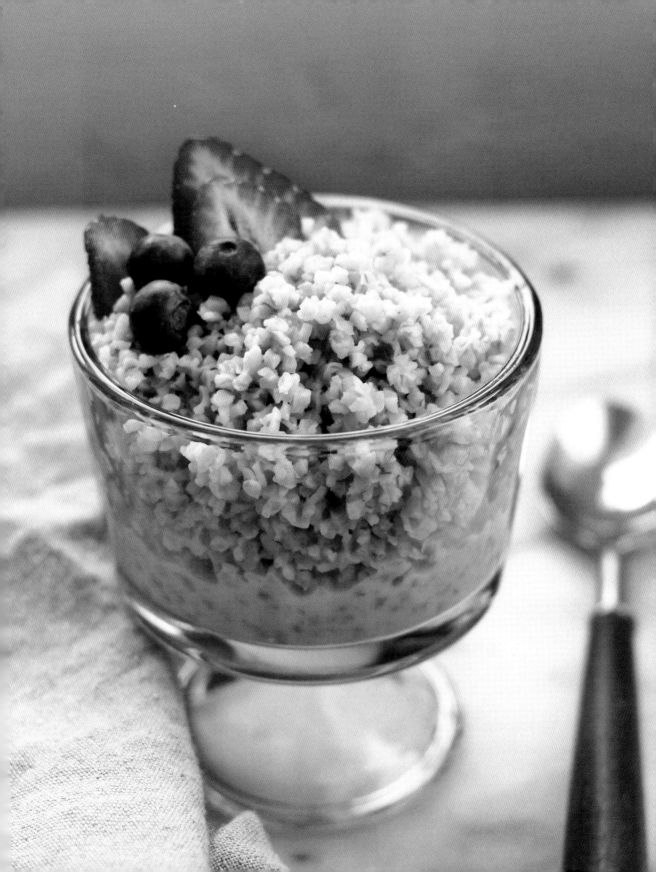

PEACH-APRICOT ALMOND BAKED OATMEAL

apricot, oats, almonds, poppy seeds

Since a bowl of oatmeal often becomes part of a breastfeeding mom's morning routine, let us introduce you to the wondrous world of baked oatmeal. Baked oatmeal has several advantages over its stovetop counterpart. It can be assembled the night before and put in the oven in the morning. It reheats exceptionally, so you can actually bake it once and eat it for several days. It is easily customizable; this version uses apricots, almonds, and poppy seeds to incorporate even more galactogogues, but you can also replace the apricots with figs and the almonds with pecans, or swap out the peach layer for slices of another firm fruit, such as ripe bananas. Have fun with it and embrace that oatmeal life!

SERVES 6

2 ripe peaches

1 ripe apricot

2 cups organic old-fashioned rolled oats

½ cup slivered almonds

1 teaspoon poppy seeds

1 teaspoon ground cinnamon

¼ teaspoon ground nutmeg

1 teaspoon baking powder

¼ cup coconut sugar

½ teaspoon Himalayan pink salt

2 cups coconut milk or almond milk

1 large egg

1 large egg white

1 teaspoon almond extract

1 teaspoon pure vanilla extract

2 tablespoons extra-virgin coconut oil, melted

1. Preheat the oven to 375°F.

2. Slice the peaches and apricot into ⅓-inch-thick slices. Line the bottom of an 8-inch square baking dish with the peach slices. Reserve the apricots for Step 4.

3. In a medium-size bowl, mix together the oats, almonds, poppy seeds, cinnamon, nutmeg, baking powder, coconut sugar, and pink salt.

4. Evenly pour the oat mixture over the peach slices. Top with the apricot slices.

5. In the same bowl used to make the oat mixture, combine the coconut milk, egg, egg white, and almond and vanilla extracts and whisk well. Pour evenly over the oat mixture. Drizzle the melted coconut oil over the top.

6. Bake for 35 to 40 minutes, or until the oatmeal has set and the top is golden brown. Serve warm. Store any leftovers, covered, in the refrigerator for up to 4 days.

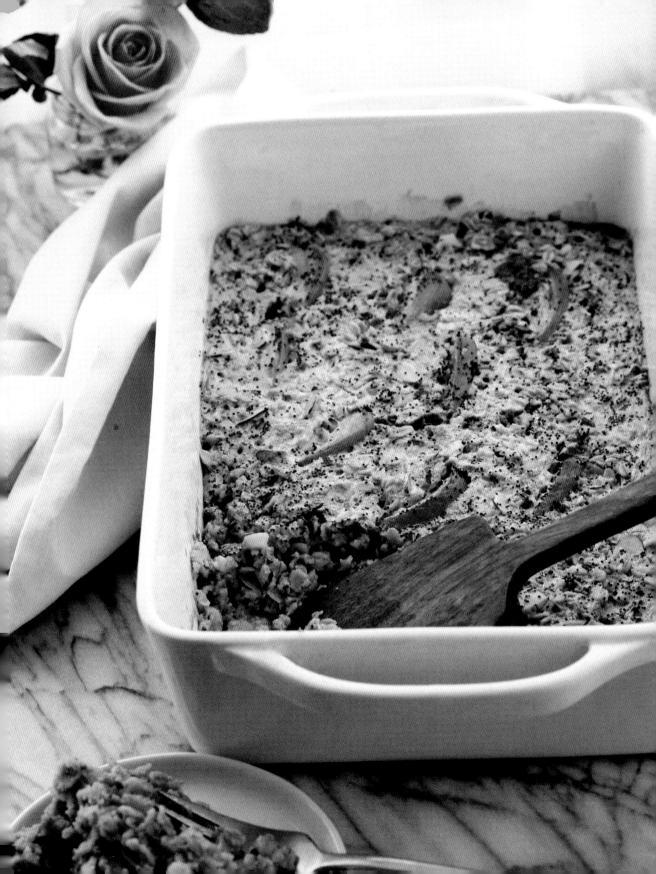

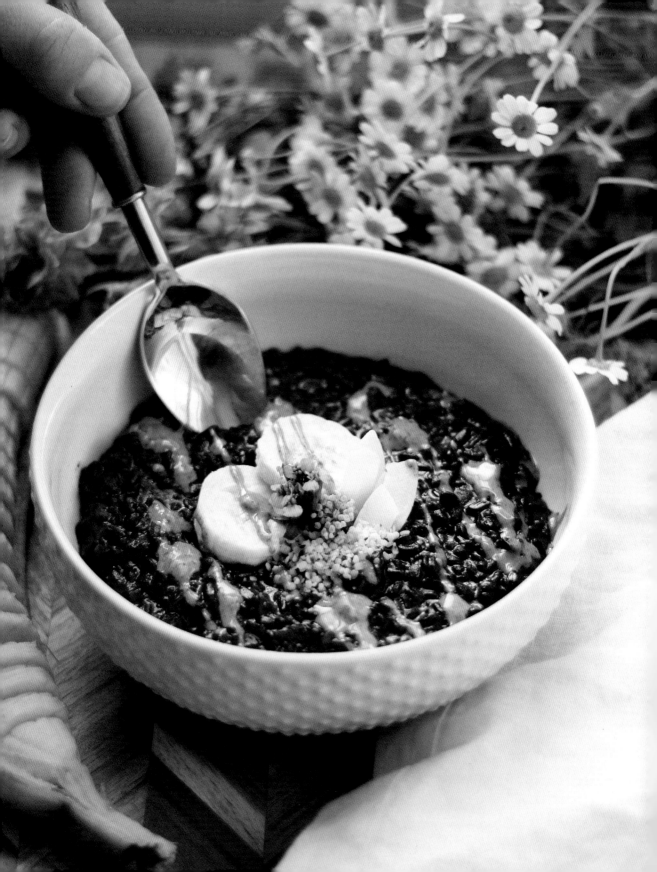

BLACK RICE CHIA PORRIDGE

black rice, chia seeds, coconut

This breakfast porridge was love at first sight—and taste. Black rice, also known as forbidden rice, turns a deep purple color with a picture-worthy glossy sheen when cooked. Its deep hue comes from an abundance of antioxidants. Adding chia seeds to this exotic superfood is a nutrient-boosting twist on a beloved Indonesian dish. For a quick breakfast prep, cook the rice the night before and store it, covered, in the fridge. Then, simply warm it back up on the stove in the morning with an extra glug of coconut milk and top with your favorites for an easy, yet luxurious meal.

SERVES 2 TO 4

1 cup uncooked black rice

1 tablespoon chia seeds

1 (13.5-ounce) can full-fat coconut milk

2 tablespoons coconut sugar

¼ teaspoon salt

1. Place all the ingredients plus 1½ cups of water in a medium-size pot. Whisk together until there are no clumps of coconut milk and the chia seeds and rice are evenly distributed.

2. Bring the mixture to a boil, and then cover the pot with a lid and lower the heat to low.

3. Simmer over low heat until most of the liquid is absorbed and the rice is softened, about 1 hour, giving a brief stir once or twice throughout to prevent sticking.

4. Enjoy warm with your favorite toppings. Store any leftovers in an airtight container in the fridge.

Suggested toppings: fresh banana slices or caramelized banana, sliced almonds, fresh or toasted coconut flakes, chunks of fresh mango, hemp seeds, splash of coconut cream, or drizzle with warm almond butter

PUMPKIN SPICE GRANOLA

oats, pecans, pumpkin seeds, brewer's yeast

Our flagship granola recipe featuring the famous galactogogue trinity: oats, flax, and brewer's yeast. Maple-kissed and baked to golden perfection, our personal favorite go-to granola is studded with roasted pecans, pumpkin seeds, and crunchy puffed millet. If you've never baked fresh granola at home, it is a life-affirming act. The warm, comforting aroma that envelops the kitchen is enough to give your milk a letdown. Sprinkle the granola on your oatmeal or smoothie, or enjoy a bowl with oat milk or mixed into yogurt. We also can't think of a more loving and thoughtful gift to bring to a new mom than a homemade batch of this granola. Deliver in a mason jar tied with a string and attach an encouraging note.

MAKES ABOUT 4 CUPS GRANOLA

2½ cups organic old-fashioned rolled oats

1 cup roughly chopped pecans

¾ cup puffed millet

3 tablespoons pumpkin seeds

2 tablespoons sunflower seeds

3 tablespoons debittered brewer's yeast

3 tablespoons ground flax

1 tablespoon ground pumpkin spice

¾ teaspoon salt

½ cup pure maple syrup

¼ cup coconut oil

1. Preheat the oven to 350°F.

2. Place all the dry ingredients in a large bowl.

3. In a small saucepan, combine the maple syrup and coconut oil and gently warm over low heat until melted, about 2 minutes.

4. Pour the wet ingredients over the dry and stir until well combined.

5. Spread the mixture in an even layer on an ungreased rimmed baking sheet.

6. Bake for 10 minutes, take it out, and give it a good stir. Then, bake for another 10 minutes, stirring it again halfway through the baking time. The granola is done when it is golden and fragrant.

7. Remove from the heat and allow to cool for up to 30 minutes. Store in an airtight container at room temperature. The granola will stay fresh for up to 2 weeks.

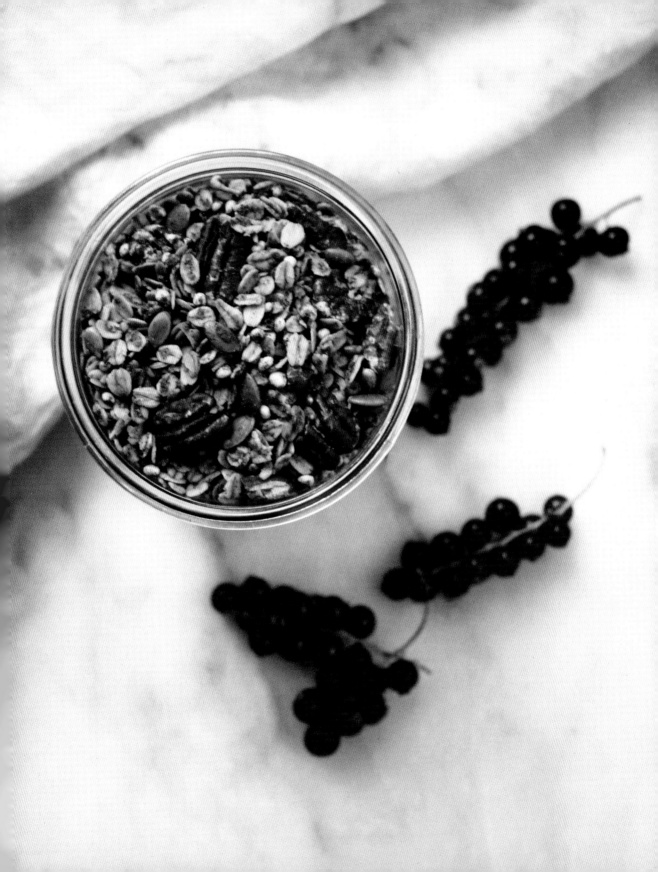

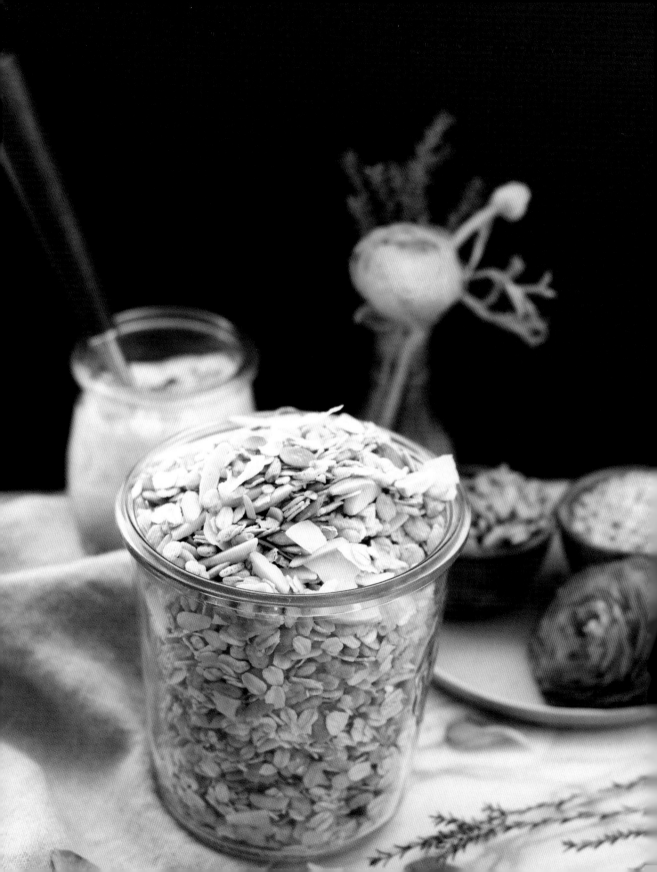

MORNING MUESLI

oats, almonds, sunflower seeds, hemp seeds, pumpkin seeds, coconut

We would never bad-mouth granola around here, but muesli does offer a few advantages over its crunchy counterpart. Muesli is made from the same delicious, hearty galactogogues as granola, but it does not contain any added sugars or oils. It is also raw, which helps keep fatty acids intact. Finally, it only takes about five minutes to mix up a big mason jar of it. You can't beat that. Spoon on top of a bowl of yogurt and honey. Soak overnight with your choice of milk. Or simply enjoy as cereal.

MAKES ABOUT 4 CUPS MUESLI

1½ cups organic old-fashioned rolled oats

½ cup oat bran

½ cup slivered almonds

3 tablespoons sunflower seeds

3 tablespoons hemp seeds

3 tablespoons pumpkin seeds

⅓ cup unsweetened shredded coconut

⅓ cup dried apple, chopped fine

Optional add-ins: dried blueberries, cranberries, or raisins

1. In a medium-size bowl, mix together all the ingredients.

2. Pour the muesli into a large mason jar with an airtight lid and store for up to a month in the cupboard.

Note: For a chewier muesli, you can toast the oats on an ungreased baking sheet in a 325°F oven for 10 to 15 minutes, stirring halfway through, until they develop a light toast. Remove from the oven, let cool, and store as instructed.

HONEY OAT CEREAL with BERRIES

oats, brown rice, millet, almonds, hemp seeds

Cereal is one of those items that many people think is best to leave to the experts and buy in a box. Not so! Not only is making your own cereal mix deeply gratifying, it's also a lot of fun and can be healthier, too. For this blend, we suggest opting for organic, all-natural, unsweetened cereals for your base, and then you can adjust the honey to your preferred level of sweetness. In our cereal, we used a blend of lactogenic grains, nuts, and seeds, to make a cereal blend loaded with crunchy, crispy bits of goodness, lightly sweetened with honey. You can't get that from a box! Once you get the basic technique down, we're sure you'll be inspired to get creative with it. (We think a maple pecan version sounds divine . . .)

MAKES ABOUT 12 SERVINGS

3 tablespoons water

⅛ cup honey

½ teaspoon pure vanilla extract

½ teaspoon ground cinnamon

4 cups oat flakes cereal

2 cups brown crispy rice cereal

1 cup puffed millet

⅓ cup organic old-fashioned rolled oats

½ cup slivered almonds

2 tablespoons raw hemp seeds

¼ cup dried blueberries

½ cup freeze-dried strawberries

1. Preheat the oven to 300°F. Line a cookie sheet with parchment paper.

2. In a small saucepan over low heat, whisk together the water, honey, vanilla, and cinnamon and heat until barely warm.

3. In a large bowl, toss together the oat flakes, crispy rice, puffed millet, rolled oats, almonds, and hemp seeds.

4. Pour the warmed wet ingredients over the dry and mix until evenly coated.

5. Pour onto the prepared cookie sheet and spread the cereal into an even layer.

6. Bake for 25 to 28 minutes, or until the mixture begins to dry out and becomes golden brown and fragrant, rotating the pan and stirring every 10 minutes to ensure the cereal cooks evenly.

7. Remove from the oven and allow to cool completely before tossing with the dried berries. Store in an airtight container for up to 2 weeks. Enjoy with oat milk or almond milk, or mixed with yogurt.

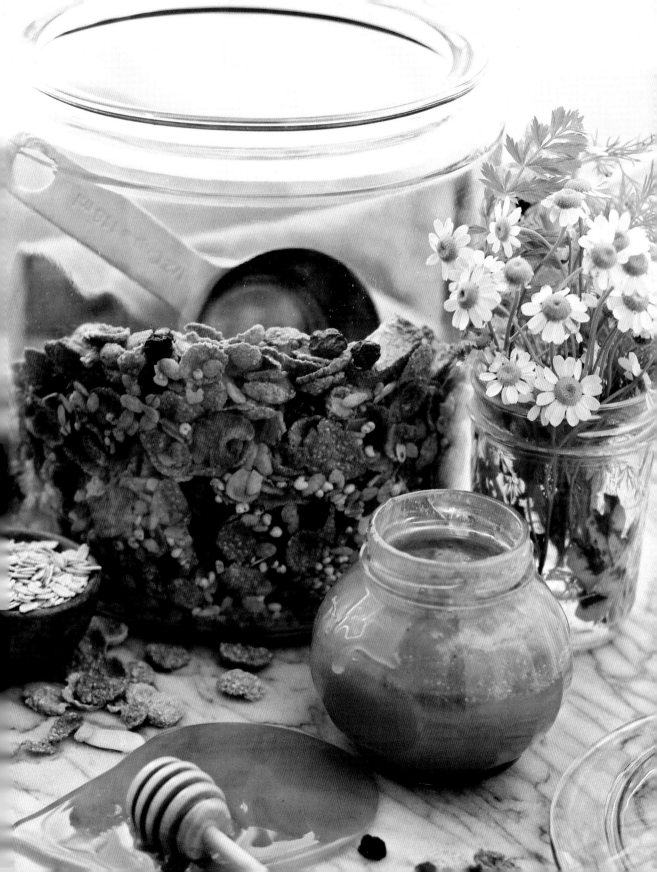

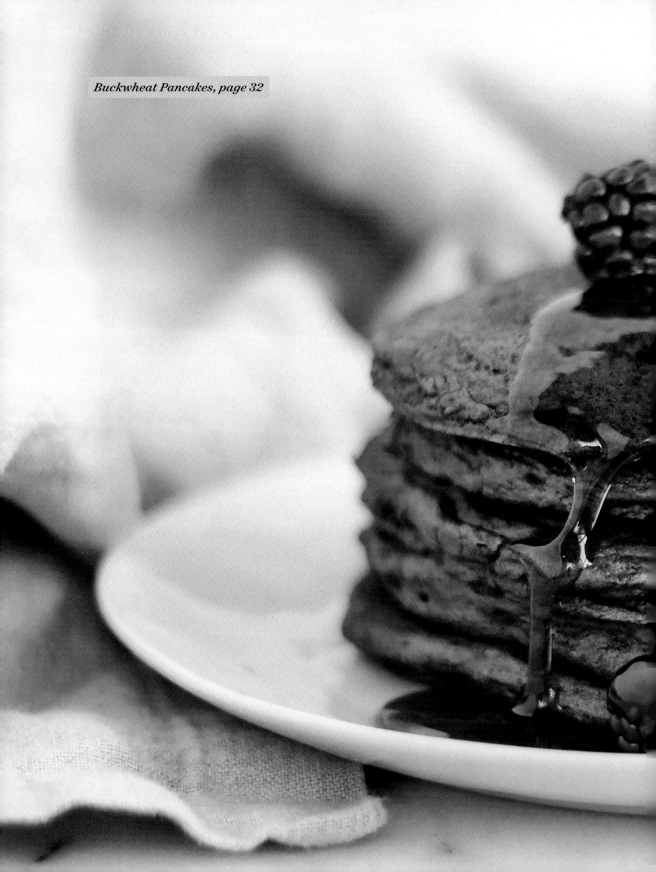

Buckwheat Pancakes, page 32

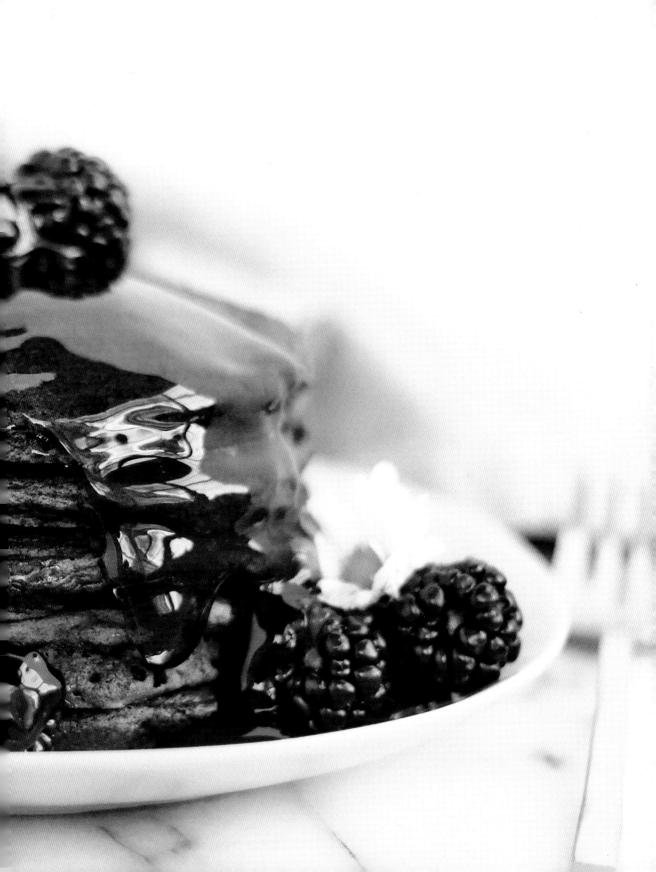

BUCKWHEAT PANCAKES

buckwheat, molasses

These buckwheat pancakes are a real surprise. It seems like whenever you try to "healthen up" a pancake, you're left with less than yummy results. Not the case with these. They are so pleasantly fluffy, yet have a deep color and flavor that is reminiscent of gingerbread. Topped with dark berries and maple syrup, they make a simple yet elegant brunch for guests coming to see the baby. You can make the batter the night before, and after they're cooked up, the pancakes freeze and reheat well, too.

SERVES 4 TO 6

½ cup buckwheat flour

½ cup all-purpose flour

1 teaspoon baking soda

½ teaspoon baking powder

½ teaspoon salt

¼ teaspoon ground cinnamon

1 cup buttermilk

2 tablespoons unsalted grass-fed butter, melted

1 large egg

2 tablespoons molasses

Fresh berries, for serving

Pure maple syrup or fresh whipped cream, for serving

1. In a large bowl, combine the buckwheat flour, all-purpose flour, baking soda, baking powder, salt, and cinnamon.

2. In a separate bowl, whisk together the buttermilk, melted butter, egg, and molasses.

3. Pour the wet ingredients over the dry and mix until just smooth.

4. When you're ready to cook the pancakes, heat a large skillet or griddle over medium-high heat until it is hot enough that a drop of water sizzles on the surface.

5. Pour ¼ cup of pancake batter at a time onto the heated skillet. Cook the pancake until small bubbles form on top and the bottom is set. With a spatula, flip the pancake to cook its other side. The pancake is done when both sides are deep brown and the pancake is cooked through. Repeat with the remaining batter. Serve warm, topped with fresh berries and maple syrup or fresh whipped cream.

CARROT CAKE BREAKFAST COOKIES

carrot, coconut oil, oats, almonds, fenugreek, flaxseeds

Who ever said you can't have cookies for breakfast? As nursing moms, we have been told how important oats are for our milk supply, but it is easy to tire of our daily bowl of oatmeal. Enter this breakfast cookie. It's not much different in nutritional value than a bowl of loaded oatmeal. If made with gluten-free oats, the recipe is gluten-free, rich in iron and fiber, and doesn't use any refined sugar. Plus, you can reach for one of these even when you're trapped on the couch with a sleeping baby on your chest. We like to top ours with a bit of cream cheese mixed with honey for "frosting."

MAKES ABOUT 15 COOKIES

½ cup finely shredded carrot

1 cup coconut sugar

8 tablespoons (1 stick, 4 ounces) unsalted grass-fed butter, at room temperature

½ cup coconut oil

2 large eggs

1½ teaspoons pure vanilla extract

1½ cups organic oat flour

½ cup almond flour

¼ teaspoon ground fenugreek

1 teaspoon ground cinnamon

½ teaspoon ground nutmeg

½ teaspoon baking soda

½ teaspoon salt

2 cups organic old-fashioned rolled oats

½ cup toasted shredded unsweetened coconut

2 tablespoons flaxseeds

½ cup raisins

1 cup roughly chopped toasted walnuts

1. Preheat the oven to 350°F and line a rimmed baking sheet with parchment paper.

2. Squeeze out and discard (or enjoy!) any excess juice from the shredded carrot.

3. In a medium-size bowl, cream together the coconut sugar, butter, and coconut oil. Beat in the eggs, carrot, and vanilla until mixed well.

4. In a large bowl, combine the oat and almond flours, spices, baking soda, and salt and whisk until evenly incorporated.

continued on page 35

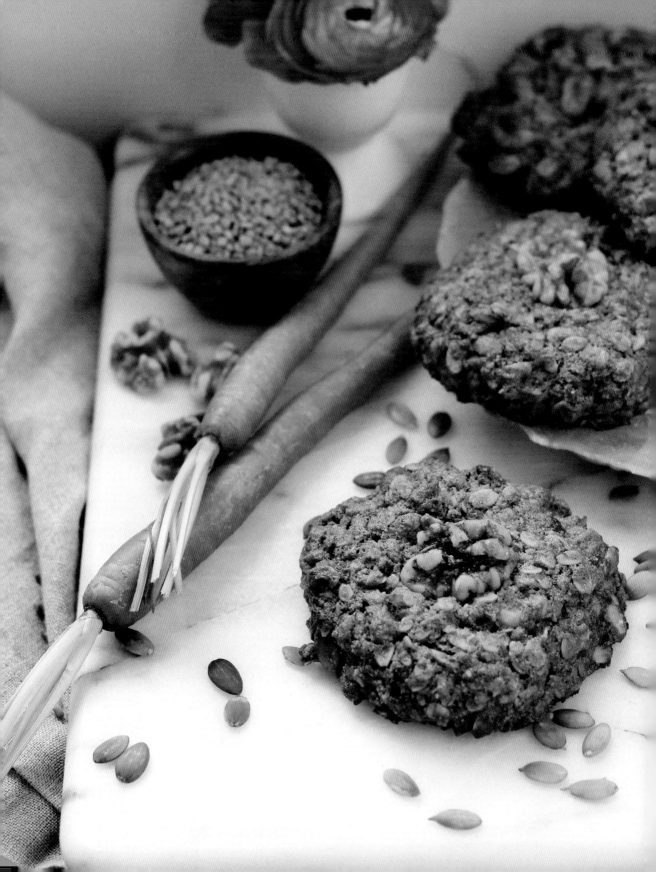

5. Pour the wet ingredients into the dry and fold together until evenly incorporated. Add the oats, coconut, flaxseeds, raisins, and walnuts. Fold until just incorporated.

6. Scoop ¼ cup of cookie dough onto the prepared baking sheet and gently flatten with the back of a spoon or measuring cup.

7. Bake for 12 to 14 minutes, or until lightly brown and firm. Transfer to a wire rack to cool. Serve warm or at room temperature. Store leftover cookies in an airtight container for up to a week.

PROTEIN WAFFLES

oats, flax, coconut

This is our family's go-to batter. It is packed with protein to start the day and is kissed with maple and cinnamon. Make a batch of these on Sunday and have them on hand for the rest of the week. They easily reheat in the toaster, microwave, or waffle iron. Is Baby eating solids? These waffles will keep him or her happily occupied. Is Baby teething? Freeze a batch of these and let him or her gnaw on them to soothe those sore gums. Have time to sit down? Top these with some fresh berries and vanilla yogurt, or toasted pecans and maple syrup.

MAKES 4 TO 6 LARGE WAFFLES

1 cup organic old-fashioned rolled oats

1 cup cottage cheese

4 large eggs

1 teaspoon baking powder

2 tablespoons ground flax

1 teaspoon ground cinnamon

2 tablespoons pure maple syrup or coconut sugar

2 tablespoons extra-virgin coconut oil

Unsalted grass-fed butter or extra-virgin coconut oil, for waffle iron

1. Place all the ingredients, except the butter, in a high-powered blender or food processor and blend for 20 to 30 seconds, or until smooth.

2. Preheat a waffle iron and lightly grease with the butter or coconut oil.

3. Pour the batter onto the heated waffle iron until it covers most of the center's surface area. Close the lid and allow to cook until golden brown.

4. Remove from the waffle iron and repeat with the remaining batter.

5. Store leftover waffles in an airtight container for up to 3 days or freeze for up to 3 months and reheat in a toaster, microwave, or back in the waffle iron.

Variation: You can also make these into pancakes. Prepare the batter as directed and cook according to the directions for the Buckwheat Pancakes, page 32.

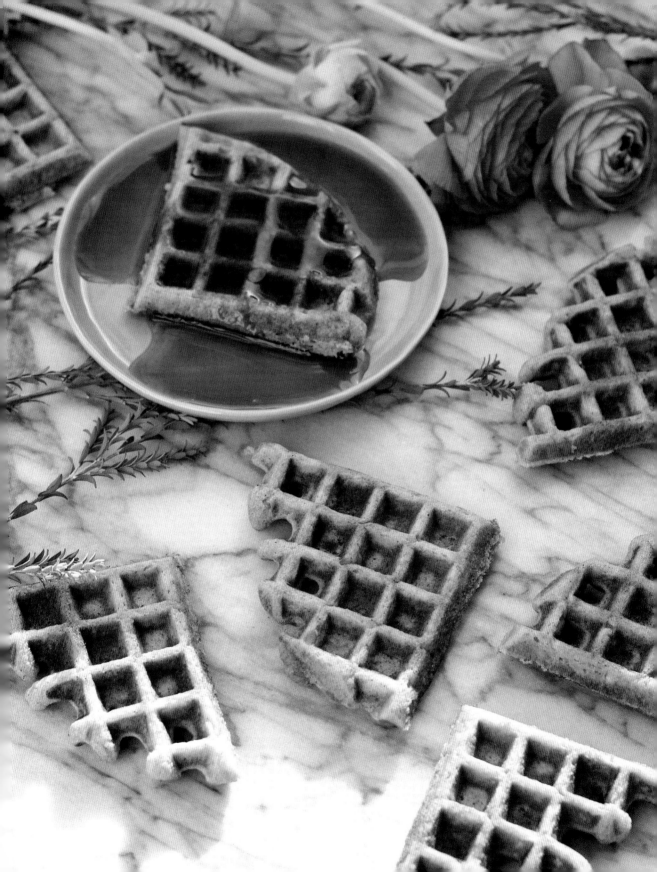

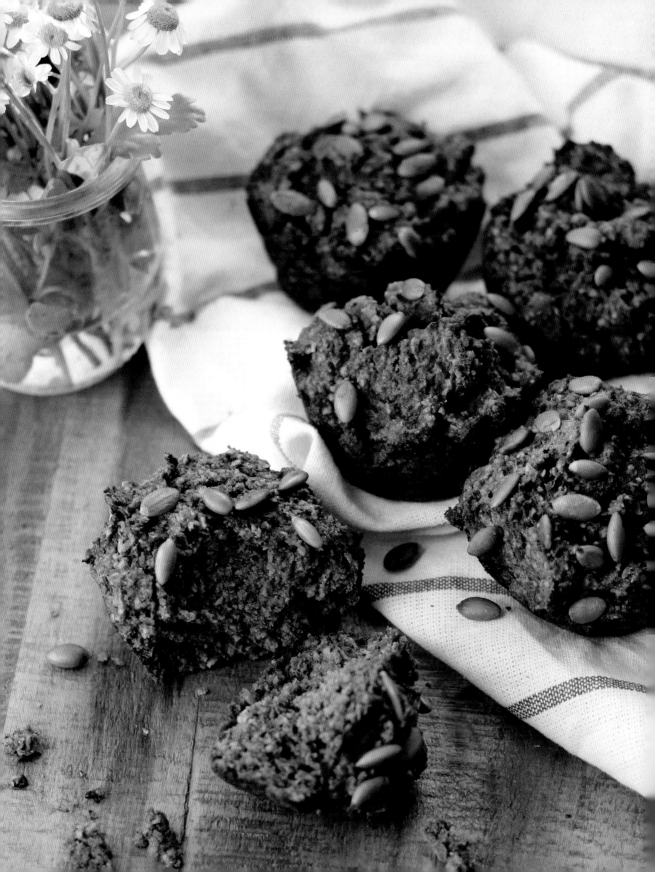

PUMPKIN OAT BRAN MUFFINS

oat bran, flax, pumpkin, pumpkin seeds

Unlike most bran muffins, which rely on a ton of oil to keep them moist, these include a can of creamy pumpkin puree. It gives the muffins an extra vitamin boost while keeping them light and moist and full of flavor. The result is a high-fiber, high-protein muffin that won't give you a sugar crash but will keep you feeling full and satisfied all morning long while you tackle your to-do list.

MAKES 12 MUFFINS

Unsalted grass-fed butter, for pan (optional)

1 cup whole wheat pastry flour

1 cup organic oat bran

¼ cup ground flax

1 teaspoon baking soda

2 teaspoons ground cinnamon

1 teaspoon ground ginger

½ teaspoon ground nutmeg

¼ teaspoon ground cloves

½ teaspoon salt

8 tablespoons (1 stick, 4 ounces) unsalted grass-fed butter, at room temperature

½ cup light brown sugar

2 large eggs

1 (16-ounce) can pure pumpkin puree

⅓ cup toasted pumpkin seeds (for garnish; optional)

1. Preheat the oven to 400°F. Lightly grease a 12-well muffin pan or line it with baking cups.

2. In a medium-size bowl, combine the whole wheat pastry flour, oat bran, ground flax, baking soda, cinnamon, ginger, nutmeg, cloves, and salt. Set aside.

3. In a large bowl, beat together the butter and brown sugar until fluffy. Add the eggs and pumpkin puree and whisk until smooth.

4. Pour the dry ingredients over the wet and mix with a spoon until just combined.

5. Spoon ¼ cup of batter into each prepared muffin well and top with the pumpkin seeds, if using.

6. Bake for 15 to 18 minutes, or until a toothpick inserted into the center of a muffin comes out clean. Remove from the oven and let cool slightly before serving.

7. Store in an airtight container at room temperature or freeze.

MORNING MORINGA SMOOTHIE

spinach, moringa, almond butter

Let's talk green smoothies. We know they've been a thing for a while now, but lots of mamas can be scared off by their alarming green color and ambitious vegetable content. And if you try going rogue and making one without a recipe, it often turns out to be a murky disaster that can turn off even the most enthusiastic sipper from giving it a second go. If you've been hesitant to dive into the green smoothie craze or have poured a few down the drain already, we're here to help. It is all about the right ratio. This smoothie packs a serious nutritious punch, but balances the "greenness" of moringa, a leafy green superfood, and spinach with the creamy richness of almond butter and sweetness of frozen bananas. Green smoothies may still be an acquired taste, but this one is worth the effort.

SERVES 1

1 cup coconut milk or almond milk

1 frozen banana

1 cup spinach, rinsed well

1 teaspoon ground moringa

1 tablespoon almond butter

Combine all the ingredients in a blender and blend until smooth. Enjoy immediately.

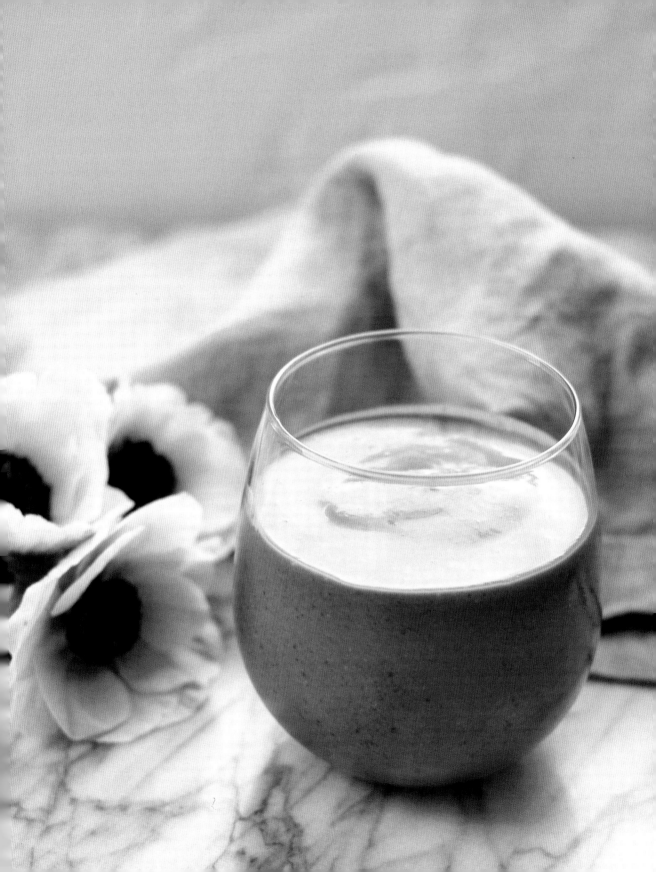

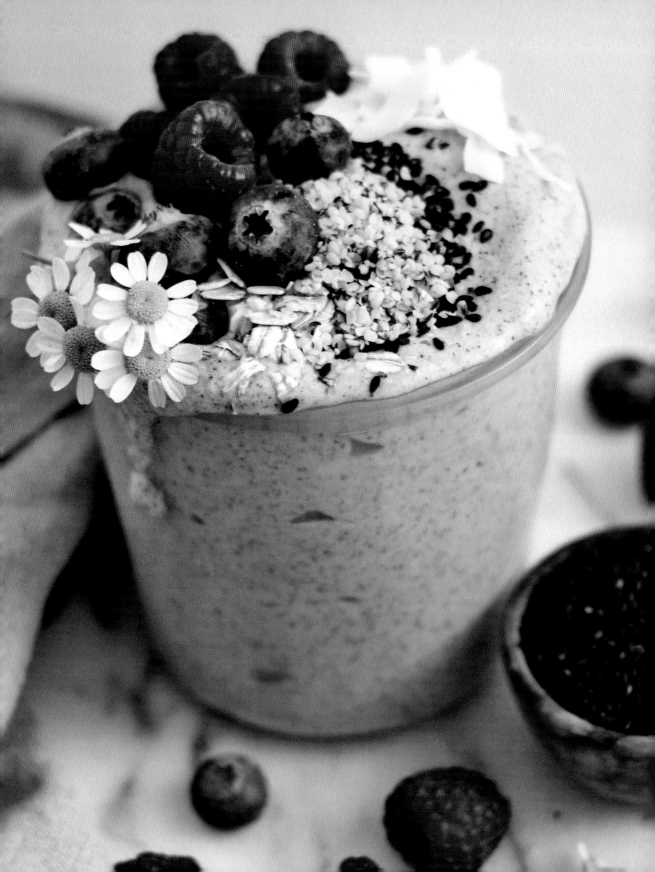

TOASTED BLACK SESAME SMOOTHIE

black sesame seeds, oats

Let's face it. Not every day is a slow, make-your-own-pancake-batter kind of day. Here's your go-to busy-morning breakfast. Unlike other fruit-based smoothies, this one adds oats to give you slow-burning energy and loads of fiber to help you feel full and tackle that early-morning nursing sesh—so it's a bit more substantial than many of the smoothies in our Drinks chapter. And if you've never added sesame seeds to your smoothie before, you're in for a treat. They impart an addictive nuttiness, similar to peanut butter, but dare we say, better. We like to top ours with coconut flakes and fresh berries.

SERVES 1

2 tablespoons black sesame seeds

1 cup coconut milk

1½ cups frozen ripe banana slices
   (about 2 medium-size bananas)

3 tablespoons organic old-fashioned
   rolled oats

3 or 4 ice cubes

1. Toast the black sesame seeds in a dry pan over medium heat for 2 to 3 minutes, or until fragrant. Remove from the heat and set aside to cool.

2. Place the cooled sesame seeds and remaining ingredients in a blender. Blend until smooth.

Note: If your frozen bananas weren't very ripe, you can add 1 tablespoon of honey to sweeten the smoothie.

Lunch

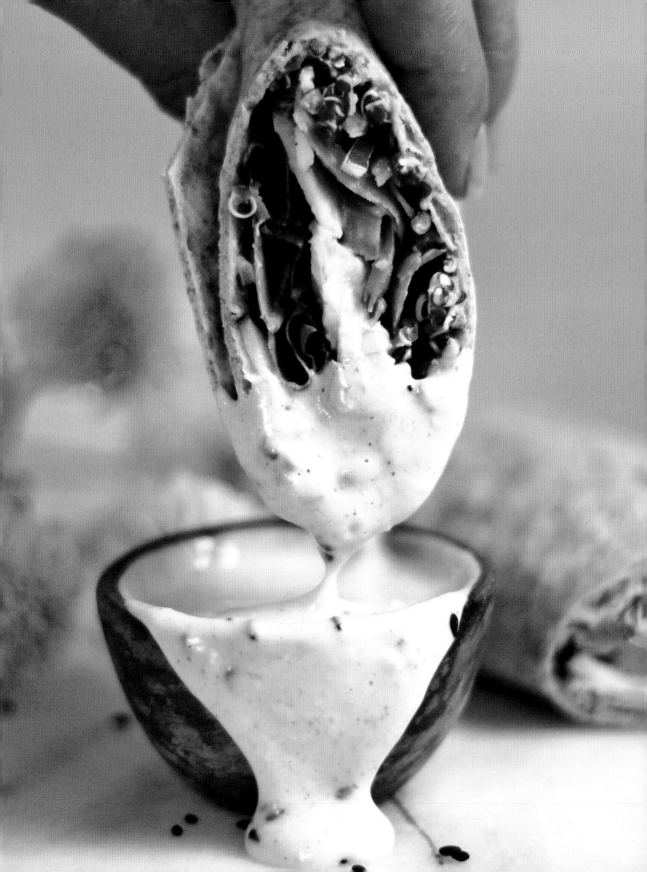

TAHINI CRUNCH WRAP

tahini, garlic, cumin, quinoa, carrot, avocado, spinach

This is a crisp, light, crunchy wrap overflowing with fresh veggies and served alongside a garlicky tahini dipping sauce. This wrap lets the vegetables speak for themselves, so try to source the freshest, organic produce you can. We find our local farmers' market has the best to choose from. We like keeping the tahini sauce and fillings separate here, instead of dressing them and then wrapping. This way retains all of the vegetables' crunch, doesn't make the quinoa or sprouts soggy, and creates an incredibly inviting and appetizing rainbow of colors.

SERVES 4

TAHINI DRESSING:

⅓ cup tahini

¼ cup freshly squeezed lemon juice

1 garlic clove, minced

½ teaspoon ground cumin

¼ teaspoon salt

½ teaspoon black sesame seeds

WRAPS:

4 pieces whole wheat lavash

1 cup cooked red quinoa

½ red onion, sliced thinly

1 carrot, cut into thin strips

1 yellow bell pepper, seeded and sliced thinly

1 cucumber, sliced thinly

1 avocado, pitted, peeled, and sliced thinly

1 cup spinach, rinsed well

1. Prepare the tahini dressing: Place all the dressing ingredients plus ⅓ cup of water in a blender and blend until smooth, about 30 seconds. Set aside.

2. Assemble the wraps: Lay out the four pieces of lavash and add the fillings evenly, beginning with the red quinoa, and then the red onion, carrot, bell pepper, cucumber, avocado, and spinach, creating a kind of rainbow. Roll up each lavash to create a wrap.

3. Divide the tahini dressing among four ramekins and use on the side to dip each wrap into between bites.

BUCKWHEAT CREPES with SPINACH AND FETA

buckwheat, spinach

While we adore crepes filled with sweet ingredients, such as chocolate hazelnut spread, they are not usually what we are craving by lunchtime. There is no reason crepes can't be for lunch, or even dinner, with this savory crepe preparation. The crepe itself has an earthy quality from the buckwheat and it is complemented by the traditional combination of spinach and feta. We added fresh peas to ours for an extra punch of protein. We can also see mashed chickpea standing in nicely. If you are new to crepe making, there is a great hack to help you get a thin, even layer. Simply pour more batter than needed into the pan, swirl as fast as you can, and pour the extra batter back into your bowl. There will be a little "tail" where you poured, but you can easily cut it off, leaving you with a perfectly round crepe.

CREPES:

MAKES ABOUT 12 CREPES

⅔ cup uncooked buckwheat groats

⅓ cup whole wheat pastry flour

2 large eggs

⅔ cup whole milk

1 tablespoon extra-virgin olive oil

¼ teaspoon salt

1 to 2 tablespoons unsalted grass-fed butter, for frying

FILLING:

SERVES 4 TO 6

1 tablespoon extra-virgin olive oil

1 red onion, sliced thinly

1 pound spinach (10 to 12 cups)

1 cup fresh or frozen peas

¼ teaspoon salt

12 ounces feta cheese, crumbled

1. Prepare the crepe batter: Place all the batter ingredients, except the butter, in a blender and blend for 10 seconds, or until combined. Pour the batter into a bowl and set aside.

2. Place a large pan (or if you have a crepe pan, even better) over medium heat. Lightly grease the pan with a little of the butter, about ¼ teaspoon. Wipe up any excess with a paper towel; the butter should not be pooling.

3. When the pan is hot, use a ¼-cup measuring cup to measure and pour enough batter for one crepe into the center of the pan. Quickly swirl the batter around

continued on page 50

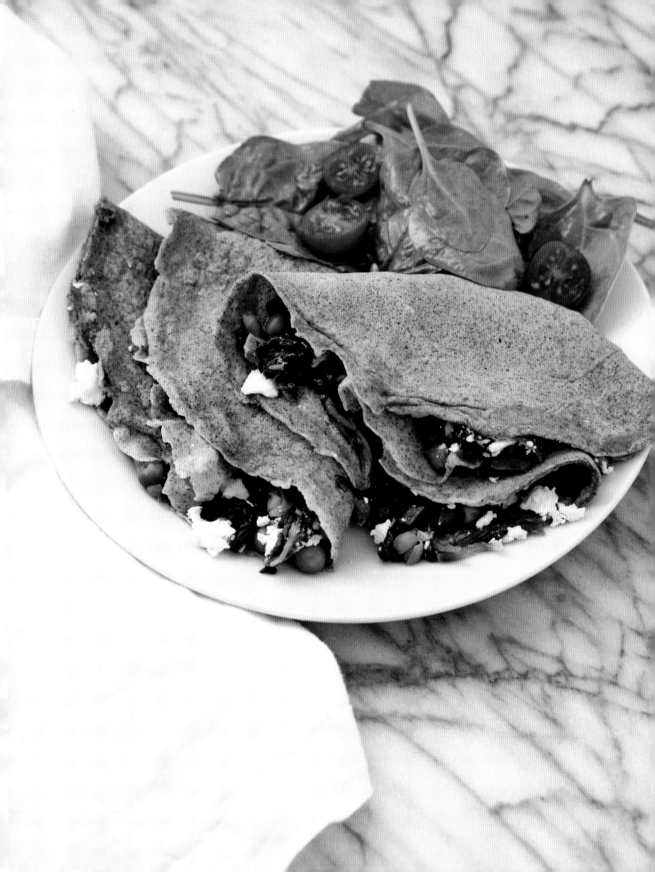

to create a very thin, even layer. The crepe should cook almost instantaneously. Using a metal spatula or the edge of a knife, gently pull up the edge of the crepe. If it pulls up, the crepe is ready to be flipped. Gently grab the edge with your fingers and flip the crepe to its other side. Cook for about 10 seconds. (Altogether, the crepe needn't be in the pan for longer than 30 seconds.) Set aside the cooked crepe on a dish, and repeat with the remaining crepes. To keep the crepes warm while you cook the whole batch, keep finished crepes covered in foil in the oven set to WARM.

4. Prepare the filling: When the crepes are finished, in the same pan over medium-high heat, heat the olive oil and add the onion. Sauté for 2 to 3 minutes, or until the onion has softened, add the spinach, and stir until the spinach has collapsed, 1 to 2 minutes more. Add the peas, 2 tablespoons of water, and salt to the pan, cover, and cook over medium heat for 3 to 4 minutes, or until the peas are bright green and cooked through. Pour the mixture into a bowl and set aside.

5. To assemble the crepes, spread about ½ cup of the vegetable mixture onto half of a crepe and top with about 2 ounces of crumbled feta. Fold the empty half of the crepe over the filling to make a semicircle, then fold again into quarters. Repeat with the remaining crepes. At this point, you can enjoy the crepes as is, or add a tablespoon of butter to the pan over medium-high heat and give the filled crepes a light fry to crisp them up, about 1 minute on each side. Leftover crepes can be stored in an airtight container in the refrigerator for 2 to 3 days.

CARROT FENNEL SOUP with DILL OIL

carrots, fennel, dill

Turning carrots into soup is a magical thing: so simple, yet so flavorful and brimming with sweetness. In a soup, carrots have a pleasant texture like that of butternut squash or pumpkin. Look for the freshest carrots you can find for the best pop of flavor—we like them just picked from the garden or bought at our local farmers' market when they are in season, but you can make this soup year-round. Depending on our mood, we sometimes leave the soup chunky and enjoy with a rustic loaf of bread, or blend until silky smooth and top with roasted pumpkin seeds.

SERVES 6

1 tablespoon extra-virgin olive oil

1½ pounds carrots, chopped

1 medium-size onion, chopped

½ fennel bulb, sliced thinly

3 garlic cloves, chopped finely

3½ cups vegetable stock

DILL OIL:

3 tablespoons chopped fresh dill

3 tablespoons extra-virgin olive oil

¾ teaspoon salt

⅓ cup roasted pumpkin seeds, for garnish

1. In a large stockpot, heat the olive oil over medium heat. Add the carrots and onion and sauté until slightly softened, about 8 minutes. Add the fennel and garlic; stir and cook for 1 minute, or until fragrant.

2. Add the vegetable stock and bring to a boil. When the broth reaches a boil, cover the pot and lower the heat to a simmer. Continue to cook for 20 to 30 minutes, or until all the vegetables are soft.

3. While the soup is cooking, prepare the dill oil: Whisk all of its ingredients together and let sit to allow the flavors to blend.

4. When the soup is done, either pour into a blender or use an immersion blender, and blend until the soup reaches your desired smoothness.

5. Ladle one serving into a bowl. Swirl about a ½ teaspoon of dill oil over the top and sprinkle with roasted pumpkin seeds.

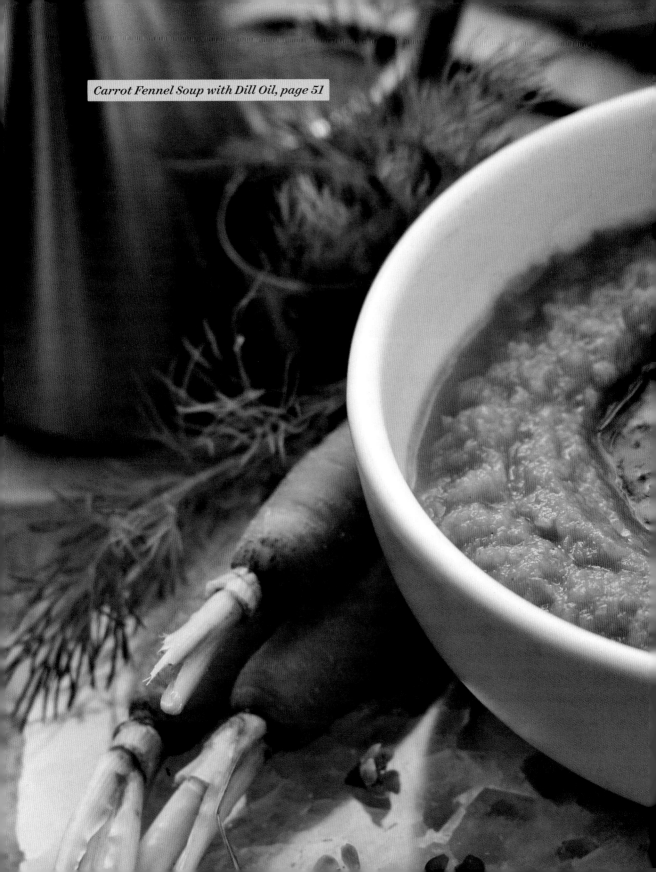

Carrot Fennel Soup with Dill Oil, page 51

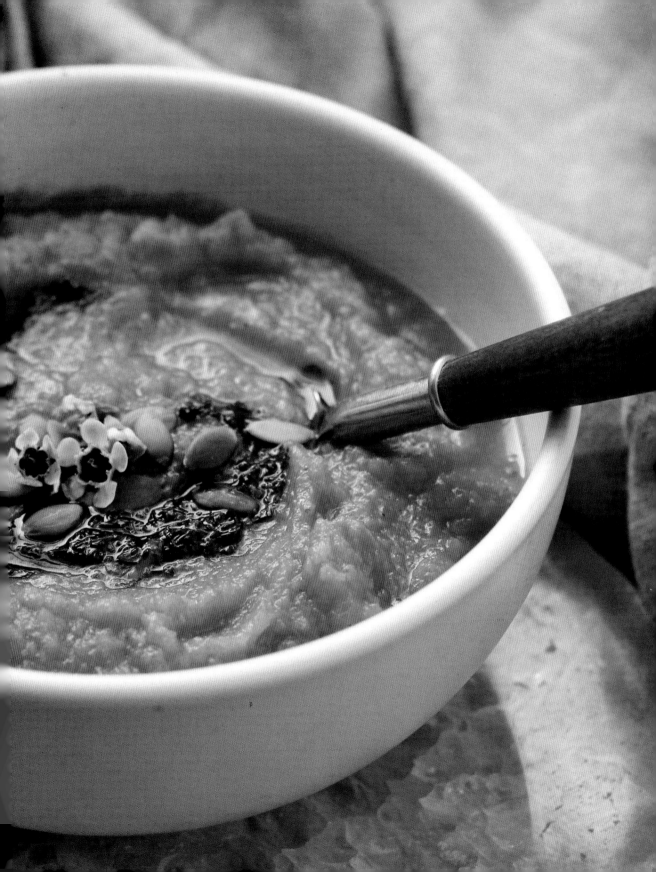

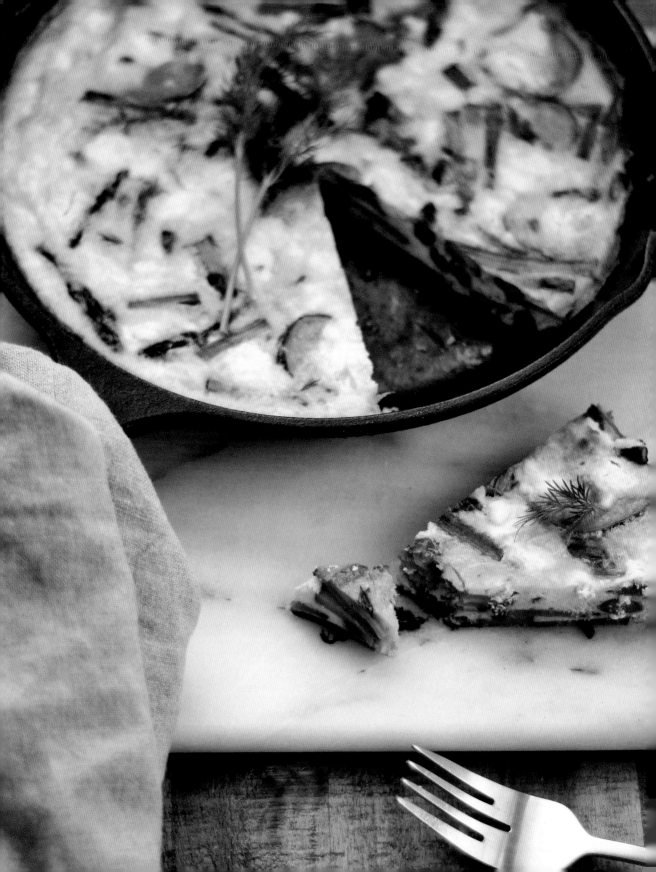

SWEET POTATO FRITTATA

sweet potato, asparagus, dill

If you don't have a few frittatas in your meal rotation, here is what you're missing: a dish that is tasty, easy, flexible, filling, healthy, and impressive-looking. You can enjoy a slice of frittata warm for breakfast and then cold for lunch. We like to cut a slab straight from the fridge and put it on top of toast or alongside a small lunch salad. One prep, two meals, supermom status. You can also fill a frittata with pretty much any vegetable you have on hand. Here we chose sweet potatoes and asparagus, and the combination is heavenly.

SERVES 6

1 tablespoon olive oil

1 medium-size sweet potato, peeled and sliced into ⅛-inch rounds

6 to 8 asparagus spears, trimmed

1 shallot, sliced thinly

7 large eggs

⅓ cup milk

1 teaspoon fresh dill, chopped

¼ teaspoon salt

½ teaspoon freshly ground black pepper

⅓ cup goat cheese, crumbled

1. Preheat the oven to 350°F.

2. In a medium-size cast-iron skillet, heat the olive oil. Add the potato slices and cook for 4 to 5 minutes, or until soft.

3. Add the asparagus and shallot and cook until the asparagus is bright green, about 1 minute more. Remove the skillet from the heat and set aside.

4. In a medium-size bowl, whisk together the eggs, milk, dill, salt, and pepper. Pour the egg mixture over the vegetables in the skillet. Top with the goat cheese crumbles.

5. Place the skillet in the oven and bake for 22 to 25 minutes, or until the middle of the frittata is fluffed up and the top is golden brown. Serve warm directly from the skillet or slice and store in the fridge for later.

KIMCHI BARLEY BOWL

barley, sesame seeds, seaweed

Kimchi fried rice is a dish popping up at trendy brunch places all over the world. Swapping out white rice for barley makes for a high-fiber, mineral-rich alternative. This recipe requires some up-front chopping and prep, but once you have all the ingredients ready to go, the dish comes together in minutes. Kimchi is a Korean fermented vegetable condiment, usually cabbage or radish, known for its healthy dose of probiotics. Kimchi has a unique and complex flavor. It is often served "raw" as a side dish, and if you didn't grow up on fermented cabbage, its pungent flavor might take some getting used to. When stir-fried, though, some of those sharper flavors mellow out and deepen, making it much more approachable.

SERVES 4

1 cup pearl barley

2½ cups lightly flavored vegetable stock or water

1 tablespoon unsalted grass-fed butter

1 cup kimchi, chopped

1 tablespoon kimchi juice (the excess liquid in the kimchi jar)

1 tablespoon tamari

Salt

TOPPINGS:

2 medium-boiled large eggs

¼ cup sliced green onion

2 avocados, pitted, peeled, and sliced

2 tablespoons toasted sesame seeds

12 sheets roasted seaweed snack, cut into strips

1. To cook the barley, combine the barley and stock in a medium-size saucepan. Bring to a boil. Cover and lower the heat to a simmer. Cook for 40 minutes, or until the barley is tender and the liquid is absorbed.

2. Heat a large skillet over medium-high heat and melt the butter. Add the cooked barley, kimchi, kimchi juice, and tamari. Sauté, stirring continuously until the barley is warmed through, the kimchi is slightly wilted, and the liquid is mostly evaporated, 4 to 5 minutes. Remove from the heat and taste. Add salt as needed.

3. Divide the barley mixture among four bowls. Top each bowl with ½ soft-boiled egg, 1 tablespoon of green onion, ½ avocado, ½ tablespoon of sesame seeds, and three sheets' worth of seaweed snack slices. Serve immediately.

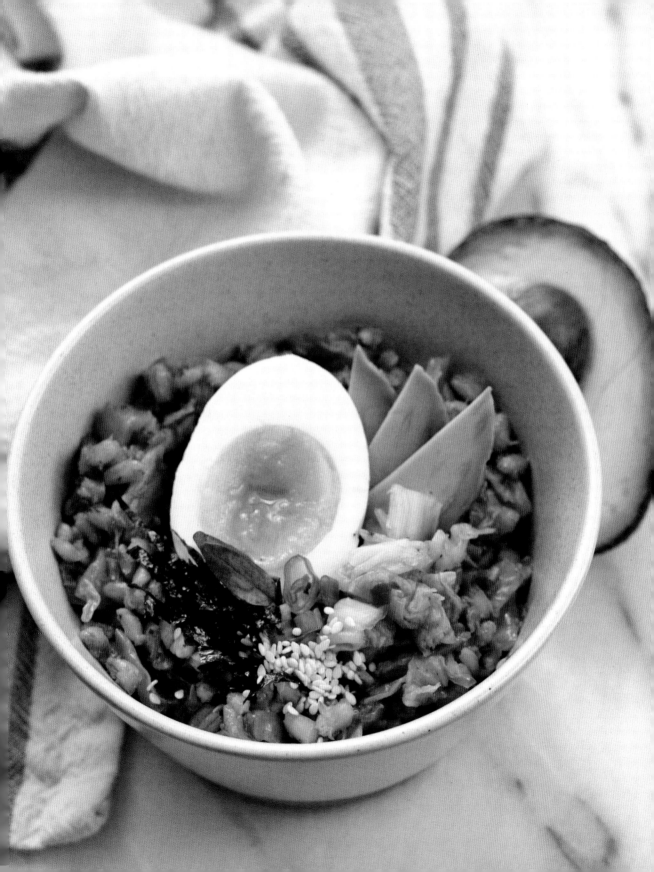

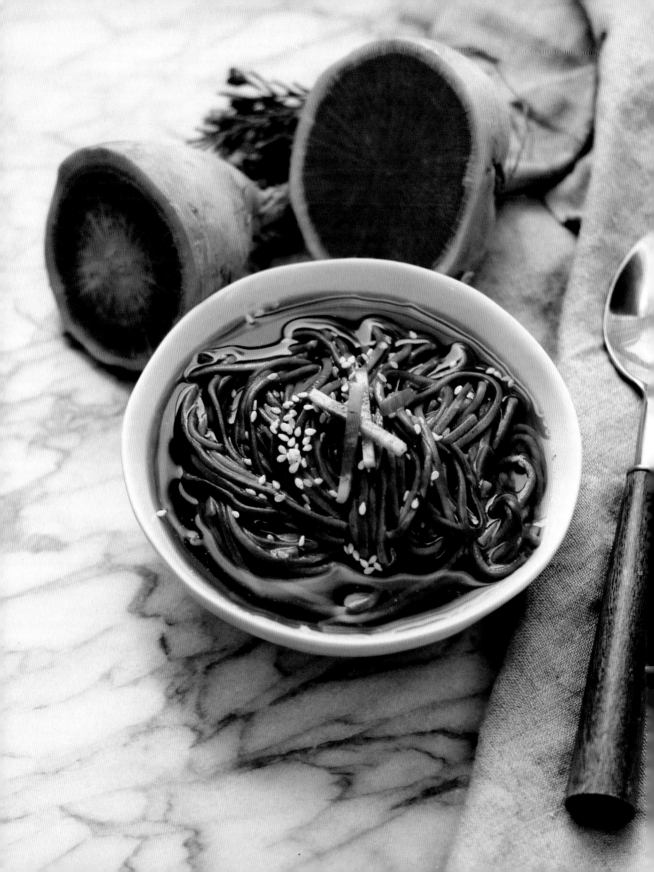

CHILLED SOBA NOODLES IN BROTH

seaweed, nutritional yeast, buckwheat, sesame seeds

You may be familiar with chilled soups like gazpacho, and you've most likely had cold pasta salad. Here is a cross between the two that is a favorite summer dish in East Asia. Traditionally the cooked soba noodles (which are made from buckwheat) are kept separate and dipped in the cold broth, but we went ahead and put them in a bowl together to make room for toppings like radish and sesame seeds. The result is a light, invigorating lunch that won't leave you feeling overly full.

SERVES 4

1 (4 by 5-inch) piece kombu

6 to 8 dried shiitake mushrooms, sliced in half

2 tablespoons nutritional yeast

½ cup soy sauce

¼ cup mirin

9 ounces soba noodles

Thinly sliced watermelon radish, chopped scallion, sesame seeds, and roasted seaweed snack, for garnish

1. Combine 4 cups of water with the kombu and mushrooms in a medium-size saucepan and bring to rapid boil. Lower the heat, cover, and simmer for 10 minutes.

2. Add the nutritional yeast, turn off the heat, and let steep for 30 minutes.

3. Pour the broth through a colander into a large bowl, straining out any big chunks. Discard the seaweed and mushrooms.

4. Stir in the soy sauce and mirin. Allow the finished broth to cool and then chill in the fridge for 2 to 3 hours or up to overnight.

5. When you're ready to serve, cook the soba noodles according to the package directions. Take care not to overcook, or the noodles will become gummy. Drain and rinse thoroughly with cold water.

6. Divide the broth and noodles evenly among four bowls. Top with watermelon radish slices, scallions, sesame seeds, and roasted seaweed snack. Serve immediately.

CRUNCHY GARLIC GREEN BEANS

almonds, garlic, ginger

The postpartum body undergoes a lot of hormonal changes, some of which can impact our digestion. This fiber-packed lunch is out-of-this-world delicious and will help keep things moving along, if you know what we mean. As is, this is a quick, light meal that delivers bite after bite of warm, gingery-garlicky crunch. To bulk it up, try the green beans over a bowl of cooked brown rice, quinoa, or barley.

SERVES 2 TO 4

2 pounds fresh green beans, trimmed

3 tablespoons soy sauce

1 tablespoon honey

1½ teaspoons rice vinegar

1 tablespoon sesame oil

3 tablespoons creamy almond butter

2 tablespoons sunflower oil

3 garlic cloves, minced

1 tablespoon grated fresh ginger

½ teaspoon red pepper flakes (optional)

½ cup chopped roasted almonds

1. Bring a large pot of water to a boil. Add the green beans and cook until slightly tender and bright green, 3 to 4 minutes. Drain in a colander and rinse well with cold water to stop the cooking. Set aside.

2. In a small bowl, combine the soy sauce, honey, rice vinegar, sesame oil, and almond butter and whisk until smooth. Set aside.

3. Heat the sunflower oil in a medium-size sauté pan over medium-high heat.

4. Add the garlic, ginger, and red pepper flakes, if using, to the sauté pan and cook, stirring constantly, until fragrant, about 1 minute, being careful not to let them burn. Add the green beans and sauté for an additional 3 to 4 minutes, stirring constantly, or until the beans are deeper green and slightly wilted.

5. Pour the green bean mixture into a bowl. Top with the almond butter sauce and garnish with the chopped almonds. Enjoy immediately.

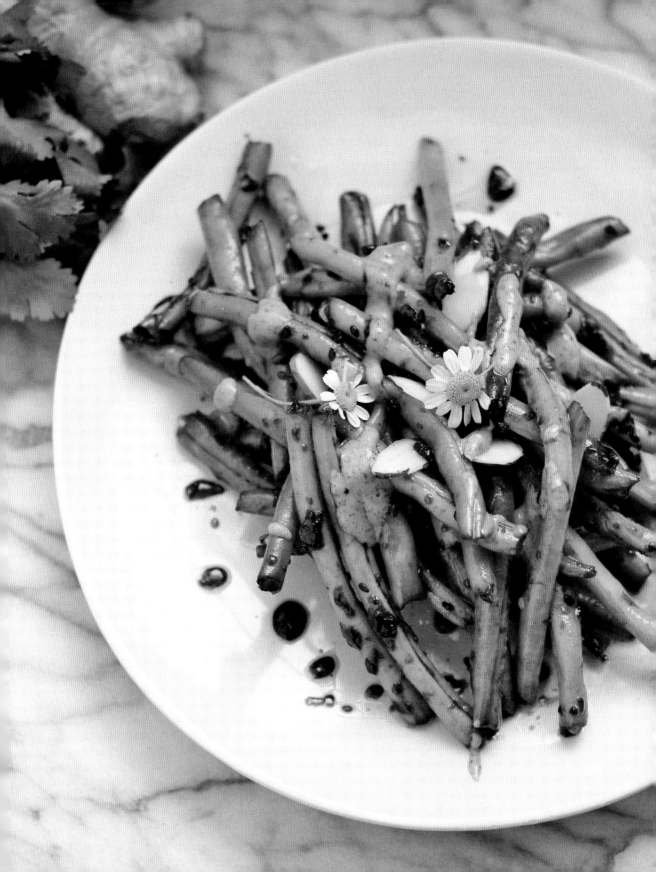

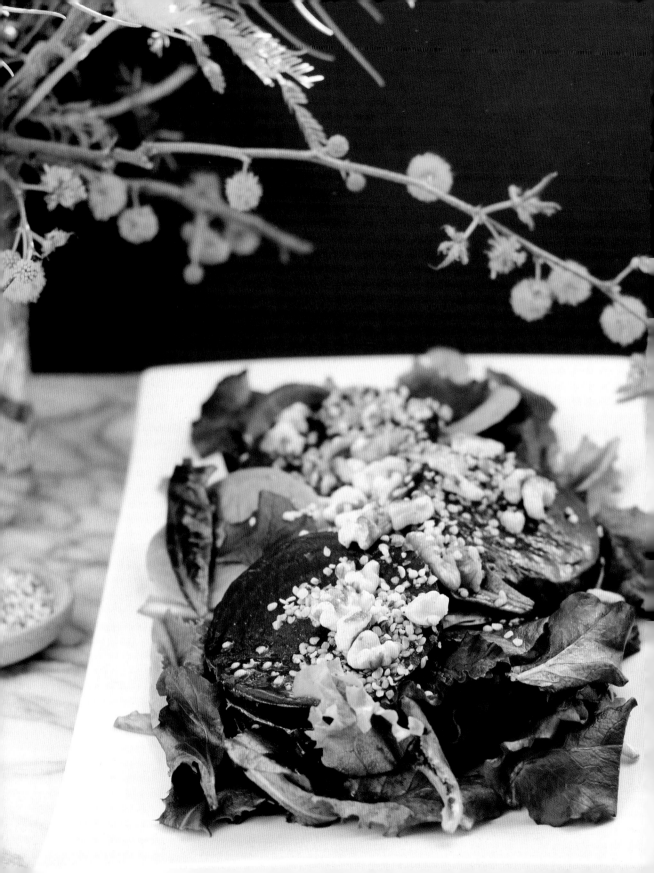

BEET SALAD with RED MISO VINAIGRETTE

greens, beets, hemp seeds

Miso is a fermented bean paste that is rich in B vitamins and helps maintain a healthy gut and immune system. Just a little bit of miso lends a deep, rich umami flavor to dishes. A touch of sweetness from honey and tartness from the vinegar create a perfect balance in this vinaigrette. It brings out the earthy sweetness of the roasted beets and mellows out any bitterness from the greens. If you're looking for more protein, you can easily add a can of rinsed white beans or a hard-boiled egg on top to round out the meal.

SERVES 1

RED MISO VINAIGRETTE:

1½ tablespoons rice vinegar

1½ teaspoons red miso paste

1½ teaspoons toasted sesame oil

1½ teaspoons vegetable oil

1 teaspoon honey

1 teaspoon tamari

BEET SALAD:

3 cups mixed greens (we like a combo of arugula, baby lettuce, baby kale, and beet greens)

2 roasted beets (see note)

1 tablespoon hemp seeds

⅓ cup toasted walnuts

1. Prepare the vinaigrette: In a small bowl, whisk together the dressing ingredients until well combined.

2. Assemble the salad: Gently toss the mixed greens with 2 to 3 tablespoons of the vinaigrette and place the greens on a serving platter.

3. Cut the beets into cubes about 1 inch thick. Place on top of the greens. Sprinkle the hemp seeds and toasted walnuts over salad. If desired, drizzle additional vinaigrette on top to finish.

4. Store any remaining dressing in an airtight container in the fridge.

Note: To roast beets, preheat your oven to 400°F. Place the beets, skin on, directly on middle oven rack and roast for 45 minutes, or until they're slightly tender and can be pierced with a fork. Remove from the oven. Let cool completely, then peel. Roasted beets will stay good in the fridge for up to a week, so you can make a larger batch and keep them on hand for salads or even snacks or smoothies.

FENNEL AND APPLE SALAD
with HONEY MUSTARD VINAIGRETTE

spinach, fennel, cashews

Did you know fennel is in the carrot family? The fennel plant is known for its sweet, licorice-flavored seeds, but fennel bulb in its raw form, especially when thinly sliced, is much milder in flavor. It provides a satisfying crunch to any salad and lends a subtle sweetness. Fennel pairs beautifully with apples and spinach, and in this salad, we top it with a zingy honey mustard dressing. This salad will no doubt make it into your weekly lunch rotation. All of its components travel easily as well, so it makes a great to-go option.

HONEY MUSTARD VINAIGRETTE:

SERVES 4

⅓ cup extra-virgin olive oil

2 tablespoons Dijon mustard

2 tablespoons cider vinegar

1½ tablespoons honey

1 tablespoon minced shallot

¼ teaspoon salt

FENNEL APPLE SALAD:

SERVES 1

3 cups spinach, well rinsed

1 fennel bulb

1 Granny Smith apple

2 ounces goat cheese

⅓ cup roasted cashews

1. Prepare the dressing: Combine the dressing ingredients in a mason jar, cover with a lid, and shake until emulsified.

2. Prepare the salad: In a medium-size bowl, toss the spinach with 2 to 3 tablespoons of the dressing, depending on your taste. Place the dressed spinach on a serving dish.

3. Cut the fennel and apple into thin slices and arrange the slices on top of the spinach.

4. Break up the goat cheese into bits and sprinkle them on top of the salad. Sprinkle with the cashews. Enjoy immediately.

5. Store any remaining dressing in an airtight container in the fridge.

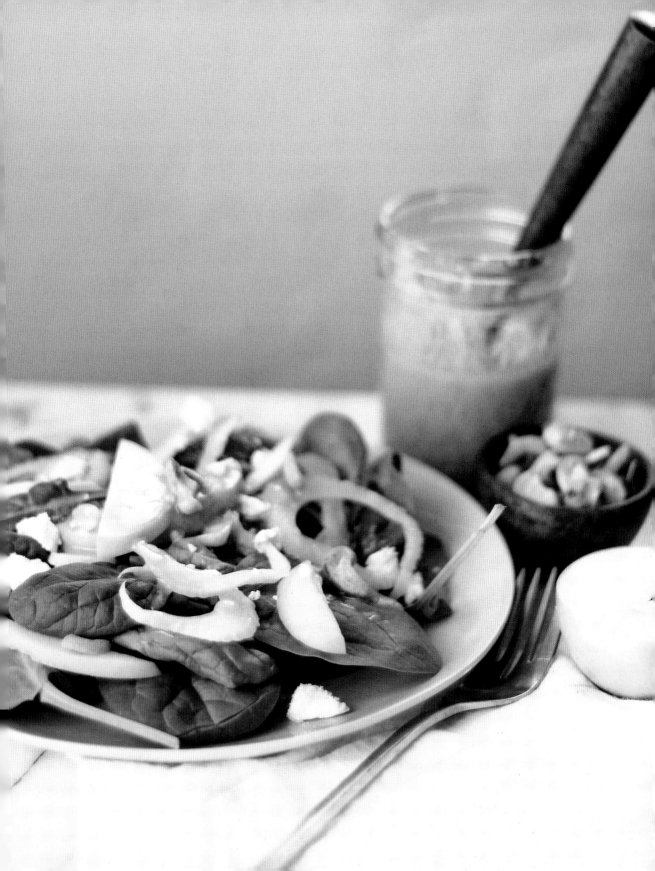

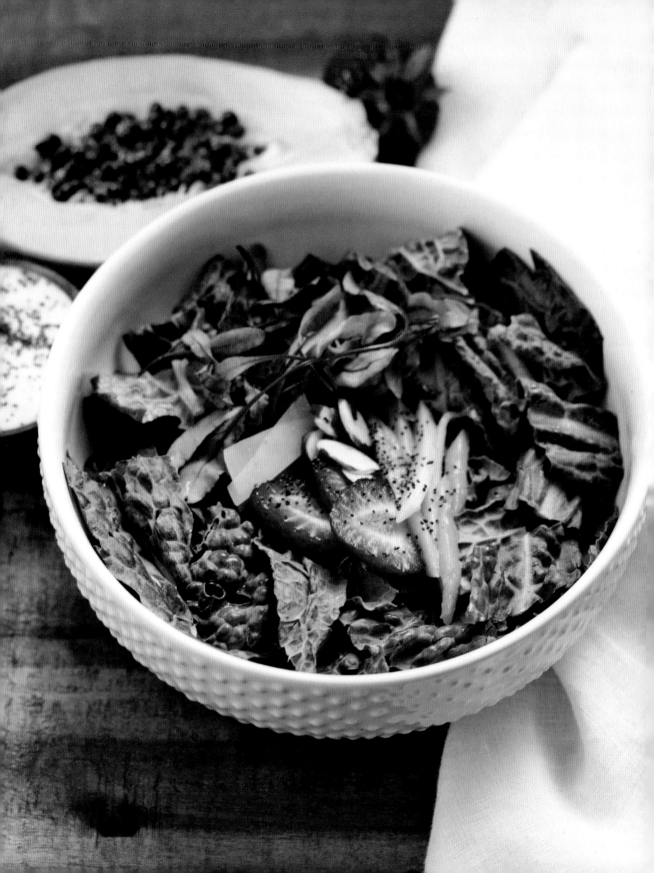

JEWEL SALAD with POPPY-SEED DRESSING

Greek yogurt, poppy seeds, kale

This salad has it all: creamy dressing, crunchy almonds, fresh kale, juicy slices of fruit, and curls of salty Parmesan. When you get a bite with a little bit of every- thing, your taste buds will jump for joy. It is a salad very rich in vitamin C, and its vibrant jewel-toned colors make it a winner for potlucks in the winter or summer. This salad comes together very quickly, and you'll even have some dressing left over that you can store in the fridge for tomorrow's lunch.

POPPY-SEED DRESSING:

SERVES 6

⅓ cup full-fat Greek yogurt

⅓ cup extra-virgin olive oil

2 tablespoons cider vinegar

1 tablespoon honey

1 teaspoon Dijon mustard

1 tablespoon minced shallot

1 tablespoon poppy seeds

½ teaspoon salt

JEWEL SALAD:

SERVES 1

3 cups lacinato kale, ribs removed

¼ cup sliced almonds

⅓ cup hulled and sliced strawberries

⅓ cup sliced papaya

1 ounce Parmigiano-Reggiano cheese

1. Prepare the dressing: Combine the dressing ingredients in a food processor and blend for 30 seconds, or until emulsified. Set aside.

2. Rinse the kale, roughly chop, and place in a medium-size bowl. Massage the kale gently with your fingers to help remove any bitterness. Add 3 to 4 tablespoons of the dressing (use more or less to your taste) and toss the kale to evenly coat.

3. Top the dressed kale with the almonds, strawberries, and papaya, and use a vegetable peeler or grater to finish with curls of Parmesan. Enjoy immediately.

4. Store any leftover dressing in an airtight container in the fridge.

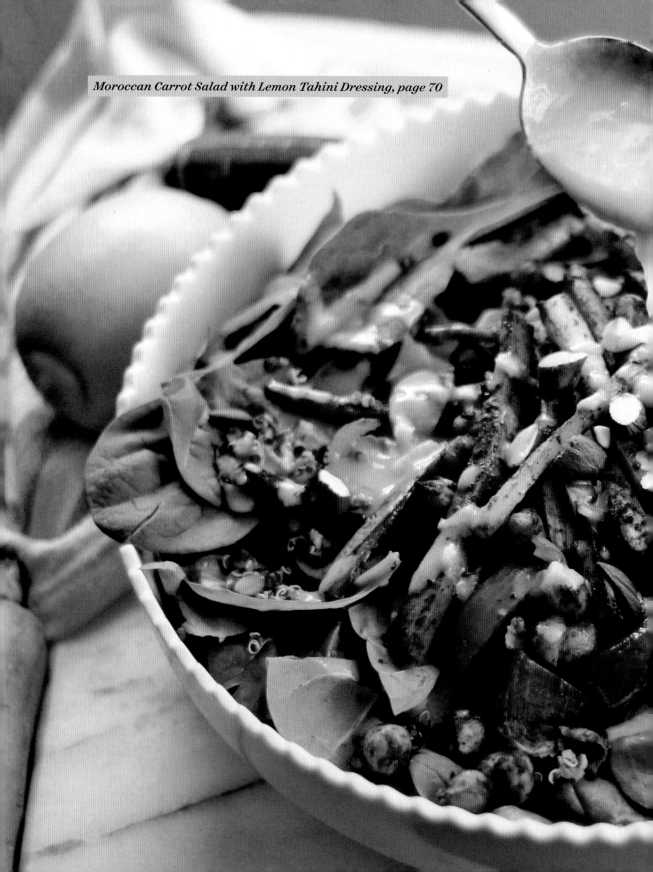

Moroccan Carrot Salad with Lemon Tahini Dressing, page 70

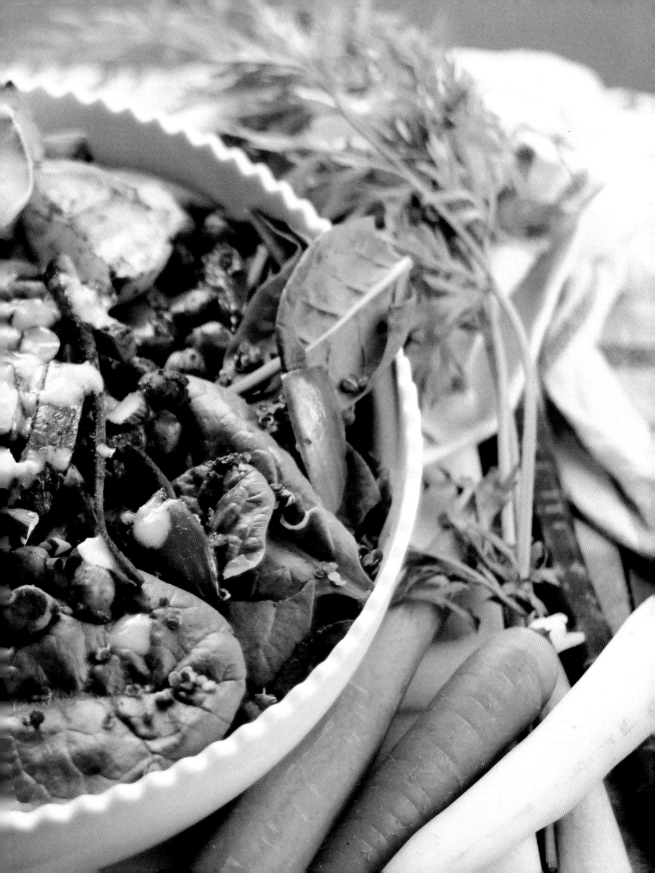

MOROCCAN CARROT SALAD
with LEMON TAHINI DRESSING

chickpeas, carrots, cumin, garlic, spinach, almonds, tahini

You might be nursing on a couch in your living room, but this salad will transport you to the bustling streets of Marrakesh. A bold blend of smoked paprika, cumin, and cinnamon complement the deep roasted sweetness of the carrots and onion. Serve on a bed of fresh spinach and toss with the creamy lemon tahini dressing.

CARROT SALAD:

SERVES 3 TO 4

1 (15-ounce) can chickpeas, drained and rinsed

8 to 10 carrots, peeled and cut into matchsticks

1 red onion, cut in half and sliced

1 lemon, cut into quarters

2 teaspoons smoked paprika

2 teaspoons ground cinnamon

1 teaspoon ground cumin

2 garlic cloves, minced

¼ teaspoons sea salt

2 tablespoons olive oil

3 cups spinach, well rinsed

2 tablespoons chopped toasted almonds

LEMON TAHINI DRESSING:

MAKES ABOUT 1 CUP DRESSING

Zest of ½ lemon

⅓ cup freshly squeezed lemon juice (from about 2 lemons)

1 garlic clove, minced

½ cup olive oil

2 tablespoons tahini

Salt

1. Preheat the oven to 425°F.

2. In a large bowl, toss together the chickpeas, carrots, red onion, lemon wedges, spices, garlic, and salt with the olive oil until nicely coated. Pour onto a baking sheet and spread out evenly. Bake for 25 minutes, or until the carrots are tender and the onion is caramelized. Remove from the oven and allow to cool slightly.

3. While the vegetables are cooking, prepare the dressing: Place all the dressing ingredients, except the salt, in a blender and pulse until smooth. Add salt to taste.

4. On a platter, spread the spinach into a bed. Top with the roasted vegetables, drizzle with 2 to 3 tablespoons of dressing, and sprinkle with the chopped almonds. Serve immediately.

5. Store any leftover dressing in an airtight container in the fridge.

WILTED KALE SALAD

beets, kale, quinoa

Here is a stunner of a grain and roasted veggie salad that is equally enjoyable warm or cold. Cold crispy salads definitely have their place, but changing up a salad with cooked components can make for a more comforting and satisfying lunch. We also like this salad because, although there is a bit of prep involved, it can all be done ahead of time and then the salad comes together in a flash. Another bonus to this salad is the roasted veggies and quinoa can easily be shared with Baby. Cubes of roasted beets and quinoa make for a fun baby-led weaning meal, or they can be zipped into a puree.

SERVES 2

2 to 3 large red beets, trimmed, peeled, and cut into 1-inch cubes

1 medium-size butternut squash, peeled, seeded, and cut into 1-inch cubes

1 large red onion, sliced

3 tablespoons extra-virgin olive oil

1 teaspoon plus a pinch of kosher salt

5 ounces baby kale, thick stems removed and discarded, chopped (about 8 cups)

1 cup cooked quinoa

Pumpkin seeds, for garnish

Hemp seeds for garnish

1. Preheat the oven to 400°F.

2. Combine the beets, squash, and red onion in a medium-size bowl. Toss with 2 tablespoons of the olive oil and 1 teaspoon of the salt.

3. Spread the vegetables in an even layer on a rimmed baking dish. Bake on the bottom rack in the oven for 20 minutes, stirring halfway, or until the red onions have collapsed and browned on the edges and the beets and butternut squash can be pierced with a fork. Remove the pan from the oven and set aside.

4. In a skillet over medium-high heat, heat the remaining tablespoon of olive oil. Add the kale and a pinch of the salt and sauté for 2 to 3 minutes. Add ¼ cup of water, cover the pan, and lower the heat to low. Steam the kale until the water has been absorbed and the kale has completely wilted and turned deep green, 8 to 10 minutes. Remove from the heat and set aside.

continued on page 72

5. To compose the salad, have two serving plates ready. On each, place ½ cup of the quinoa, then half of the wilted kale, then half of the roasted beets, squash, and onion, and top with pumpkin and hemp seeds. Finish with a drizzle of extra-virgin olive oil.

Note: For this salad, we prefer to cook our quinoa in vegetable stock instead of water, for added flavor. Also, we used tricolor quinoa, but any color will do.

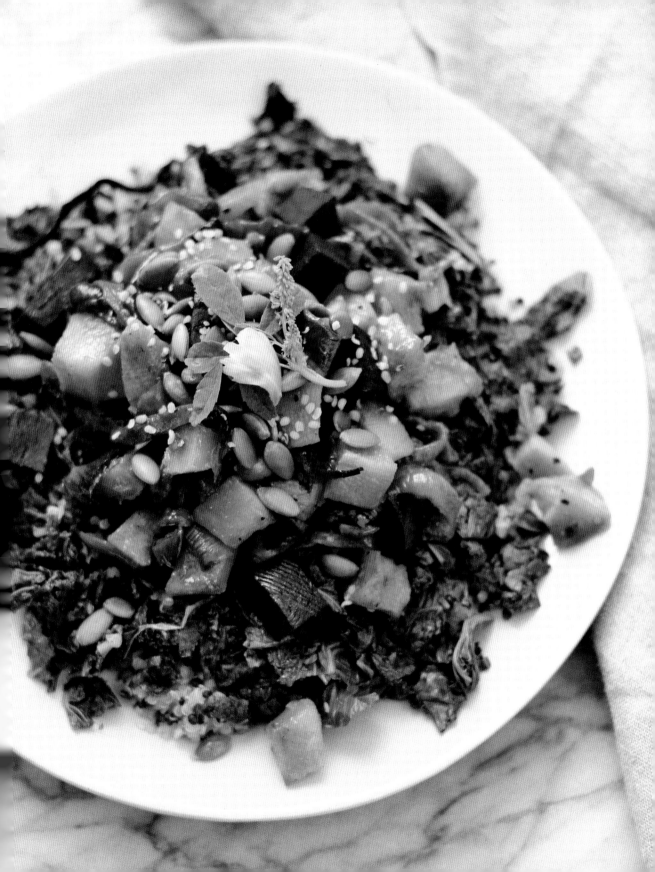

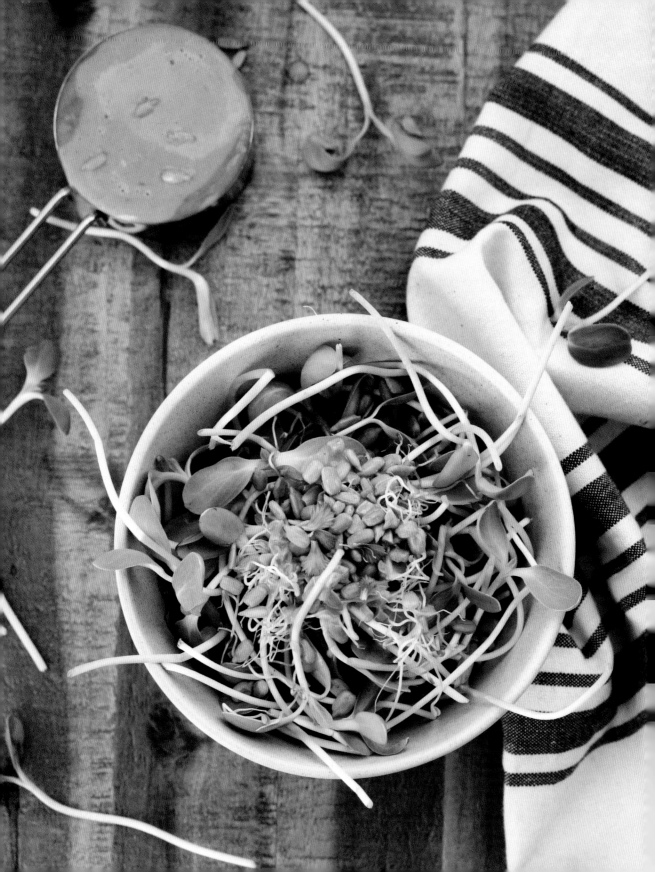

SPROUTED SALAD with SUNFLOWER DRESSING

sunflower seeds, ginger, garlic, fenugreek

We've seen peanut butter dressings and tahini dressings, so we thought, how about a sunflower seed butter dressing? And it did not disappoint. The sunflower seed butter makes such a creamy, nutty, slightly sweet dressing. Together with a mixture of fresh sprouts, it creates this simple salad that will make your taste buds sing. It is a recipe we continue to come back to time and again. Enjoy as is as a light lunch or top with a hard-boiled egg or chickpeas for extra protein.

SUNFLOWER DRESSING:

SERVES 6

¼ cup sunflower seed butter

2 tablespoons extra-virgin olive oil

1 tablespoon honey

1 tablespoon soy sauce

1 tablespoon rice vinegar

1 tablespoon freshly squeezed lime juice

1 teaspoon grated fresh ginger

1 garlic clove, smashed

3 tablespoons warm water, plus more if needed

SPROUTED SALAD:

SERVES 1

1 cup sunflower seed sprouts

¼ cup clover sprouts

¼ cup fenugreek sprouts

2 tablespoons roasted, unsalted sunflower seeds

1. Prepare the dressing: Combine all the dressing ingredients in a food processor and pulse for 30 seconds, or until smooth and creamy. If the dressing is too thick, add a little more warm water to loosen it.

2. Prepare the salad: Mix together the fresh sprouts in a bowl. Toss gently with 2 to 3 tablespoons of the dressing (or more to taste) and top with the sunflower seeds.

3. Store any leftover dressing in an airtight container in the fridge.

SUNSHINE FRITTERS

beet, carrots, kale, dill

Give me all the savory patties, cakes, and fritters, please. The centers of these remain warm and soft, while the outsides get crisp and the edges of the veggies get a bit fried. (Those are the best bits!) These fritters are so versatile. Serve them on a bed of greens or top them with our Veggie Dill Dip (page 102) for a tasty vegetable-packed lunch. Watch out, because nearby toddlers will devour these hot off the pan . . .

MAKES ABOUT 12 FRITTERS

- 1 medium-size golden beet, peeled and shredded (about 1 cup)
- 2 medium-size carrots, peeled into ribbons (about 1 cup)
- 7 to 8 lacinato kale leaves, stemmed and sliced into ribbons (about 1 cup)
- ¼ red onion, peeled and sliced thinly (about ½ cup)
- 1 tablespoon chopped fresh dill
- ¼ cup all-purpose flour
- ½ teaspoon kosher salt
- 3 large eggs, lightly beaten
- About 2 tablespoons canola or peanut oil, for frying

1. Place all the vegetables and dill in a large bowl. Pour the flour and salt over them and toss until evenly coated.

2. Pour the beaten eggs over the vegetables and mix until coated.

3. Place a large skillet over medium-high heat. Add your frying oil of choice and heat.

4. Fill a ¼-cup measure with the vegetable mixture and drop the contents into the hot oil, immediately spreading it out into a patty with about a ½-inch thickness.

5. Cook for about 3 minutes, or until the edges start to brown, then flip with a large spatula. Cook for another 1 to 2 minutes. The underside should be lightly browned.

6. Remove the fritter from the pan and place on a clean paper towel. Or place it on a cookie sheet and hold in a warm oven until the rest of the fritters are done. Prepare the remaining fritters. Serve immediately.

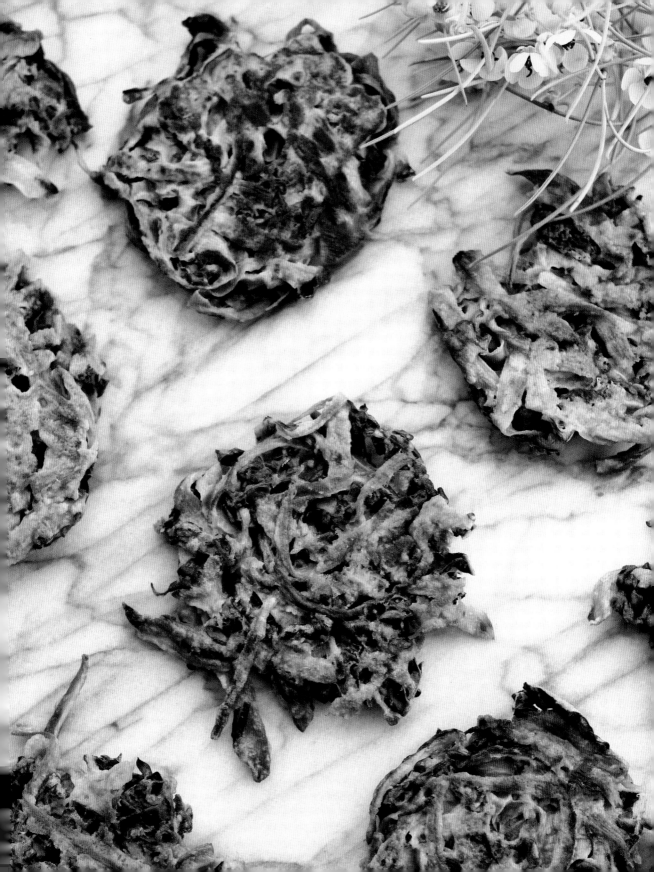

Snacks

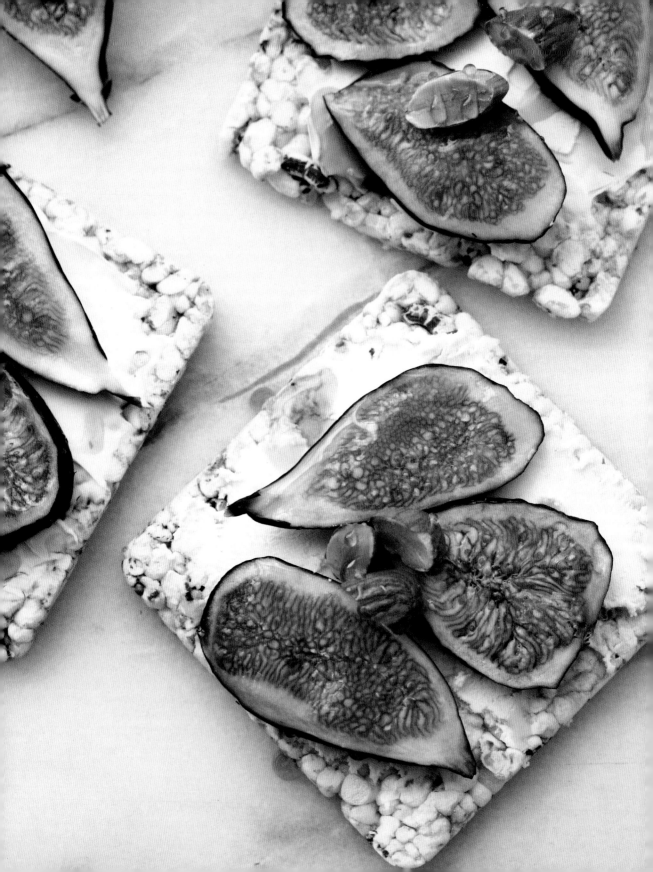

FIG-GOAT CHEESE RICE CAKES

brown rice, figs, almonds, hemp seeds

These little bites are almost too pretty to eat . . . almost. When fresh figs are in season, we are the first in line at the local farmers' market. We used fresh Black Mission figs here, but you can also substitute dried when fresh are not available. Figs pair beautifully with the slightly salty profile of goat cheese and the rice cakes and nuts deliver a contrasting crunch. Drizzle with a little raw honey, and you have a snack that will satisfy all of your cravings and deliver a ton of antioxidants.

SERVES 1

2 tablespoons goat cheese

2 thin brown rice cakes

1 fresh fig, sliced thinly

1 tablespoon chopped roasted almonds

½ teaspoon hemp seeds

Honey, for topping (optional)

Spread the goat cheese evenly on the rice cakes and layer it with thin slices of fig, the chopped almonds, the hemp seeds, and a light drizzle of honey, if using. Enjoy immediately.

BLUEBERRY WALNUT OAT BITES

coconut oil, oats, brewer's yeast, sunflower seeds, black sesame seeds, flaxseeds, hemp seeds, chia seeds

These oat bites are like a cross between a muffin and an oatmeal cookie. They are very hearty and filling and won't get smushed in your diaper bag. The seed blend in these helps deliver trace minerals, protein, and omega-3s to keep you energized.

MAKES 12 BARS

Coconut oil or unsalted grass-fed butter, for pan

⅔ cup extra-virgin coconut oil

¾ cup honey

3 cups organic old-fashioned rolled oats

1¾ cups organic oat flour

2 tablespoons debittered brewer's yeast

2 teaspoons Himalayan pink salt

½ teaspoon aluminum-free baking powder

¾ cup chopped walnuts

¼ cup roasted unsalted sunflower seeds

2 tablespoons black sesame seeds

3 tablespoons flaxseeds

1 tablespoon hemp seeds

1 tablespoons chia seeds

½ teaspoon ground cinnamon

½ cup coconut sugar

½ cup dried blueberries

2 large eggs, lightly beaten

1. Place the oven rack at the top third of the oven and preheat the oven to 325°F. Grease a 12-well muffin pan with coconut oil or butter.

2. In a medium-size saucepan over low heat, melt the coconut oil. Next, stir in the honey until just warm. Do not bring to a boil.

3. In a large bowl, combine all the remaining ingredients, except the eggs, and mix well.

4. Pour the warm honey mixture over the dry ingredients and mix until just combined. Slowly stir in the beaten eggs until the batter comes together. Do not overmix.

5. Scoop the batter evenly into the prepared muffin wells, pressing gently down on each one, and bake for 25 to 30 minutes, or until a toothpick inserted into the center of a muffin comes out clean.

6. Remove from the oven and allow to cool for 10 minutes before removing from the pan. Store in an airtight container for up to a week.

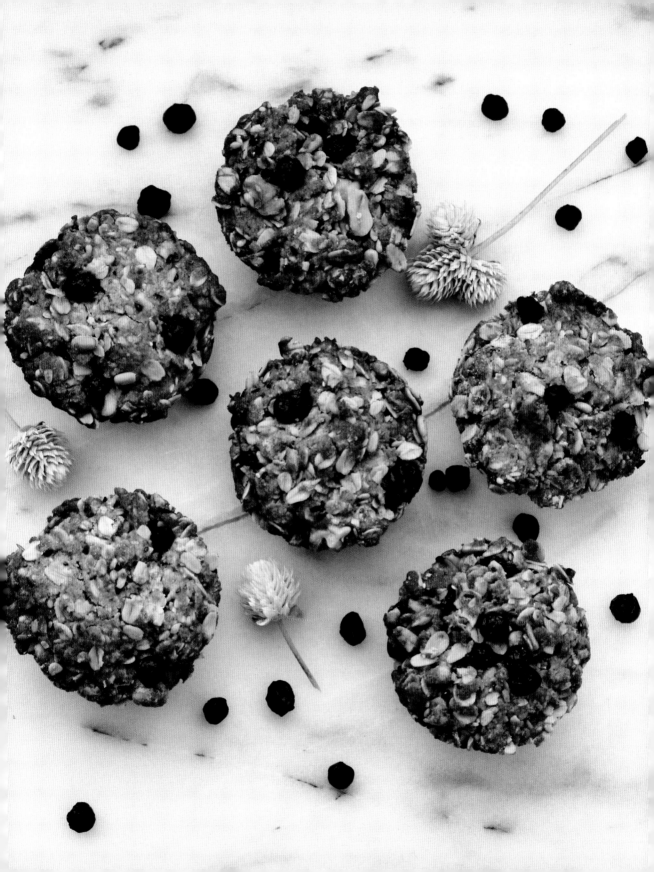

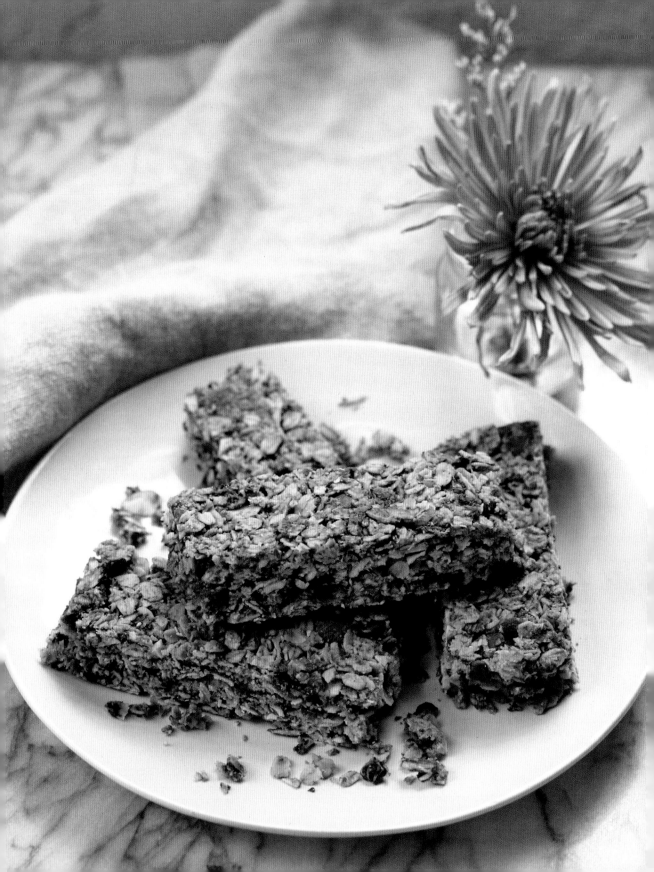

LACTATION GRANOLA BARS

oats, brewer's yeast, flax, coconut, almonds, chia seeds

What better delivery system of the lactation trio of oats, flax, and brewer's yeast than a chewy granola bar? After all, tasty bars like this are what our company is known for. Toasting the dry ingredients lends that signature golden brown, toasty goodness, and helps mellow out any bitterness from the yeast. Pack them in your diaper bag, or store them beside your nursing chair for when breastfeeding hunger strikes.

MAKES 12 BARS

2 cups organic old-fashioned rolled oats

2 tablespoons debittered brewer's yeast

⅓ cup ground flax

1 cup unsweetened shredded coconut

1 cup slivered almonds

1 teaspoon chia seeds

6 pitted dates, chopped

¼ cup coconut sugar

⅔ cup pure maple syrup

3 tablespoons coconut oil

1½ teaspoons pure vanilla extract

¼ teaspoon salt

¼ cup semisweet chocolate chips or dried fruit

1. Preheat the oven to 325°F.

2. Combine the oats, brewer's yeast, ground flax, coconut, and almonds on an ungreased cookie sheet. Spread out evenly and bake for 10 minutes, or until lightly toasted. Remove from the oven. Lower the oven temperature to 300°F. Line an 8-inch square baking pan with parchment paper and set aside.

3. In a large bowl, add the toasted ingredients, chia seeds, dates, and coconut sugar.

4. In a small saucepan, bring the maple syrup, coconut oil, vanilla, and salt to a low boil and simmer for 2 minutes.

5. Pour over the dry ingredients and mix until fully incorporated.

6. Quickly stir in the chocolate chips and pour into the prepared baking pan, spreading out evenly. Use a piece of wax paper to press down firmly to flatten.

7. Bake for 25 to 30 minutes at 300°F, or until the edges are golden brown.

8. Remove from the oven and allow to cool for 1 hour before removing from the pan to cut. Cut into twelve bars and store in an airtight container for up to 2 weeks.

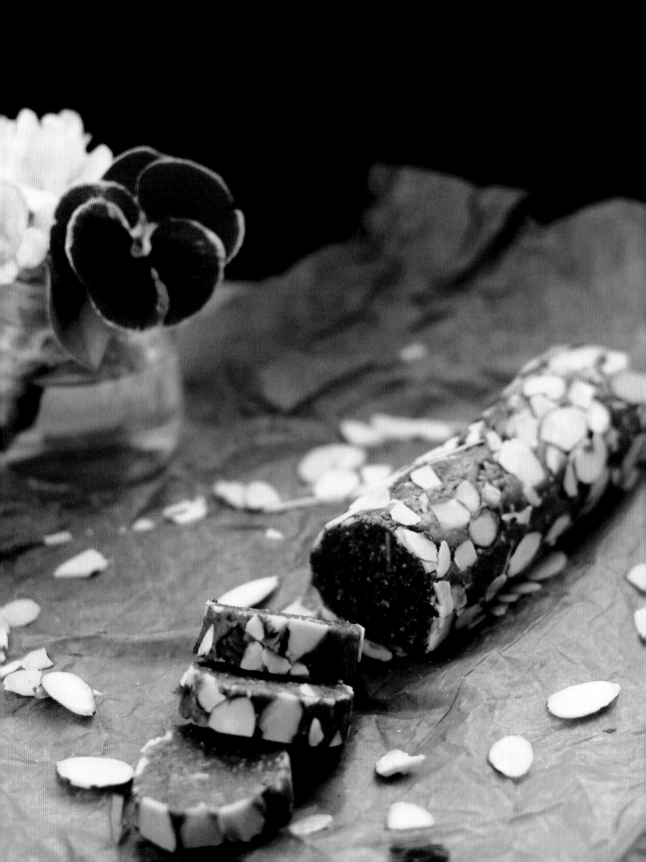

NO-BAKE FIG COOKIES

dried figs, almonds, cashews, oats, coconut oil

The chewiness of the oats, the crunch of the almonds, the natural sun-ripened sweetness of the figs, and the hint of orange make these not your average no-bake cookie. Friends have described them as raw Fig Newtons. Without any added sugars or white flours, you can feel great (and sneaky) about sharing these with cookie-loving toddlers. That is, if you'll have any left to share.

MAKES 12 COOKIES

1½ cups dried golden figs

1½ cups water or orange juice

½ cup raw almonds

½ cup raw cashews

½ cup organic quick-cooking oats

2 tablespoons virgin coconut oil

½ teaspoon ground cinnamon

½ teaspoon orange oil

¼ teaspoon salt

½ cup sliced almonds, for rolling

1. Place the figs in the water or orange juice and let soak for 5 minutes. Drain the liquid.

2. Place the soaked figs and the remaining ingredients in a high-powered blender or food processor and pulse until a sticky ball forms.

3. Remove the "dough" from the food processor and place on a long piece of waxed paper. Form the dough into a log and roll in the sliced almonds. Wrap the log in the waxed paper and refrigerate for 1 hour or overnight.

4. Remove from the refrigerator and slice into disks about ½ inch thick. Store the cookies in an airtight container in the fridge, separated by pieces of waxed or parchment paper to prevent them from sticking together.

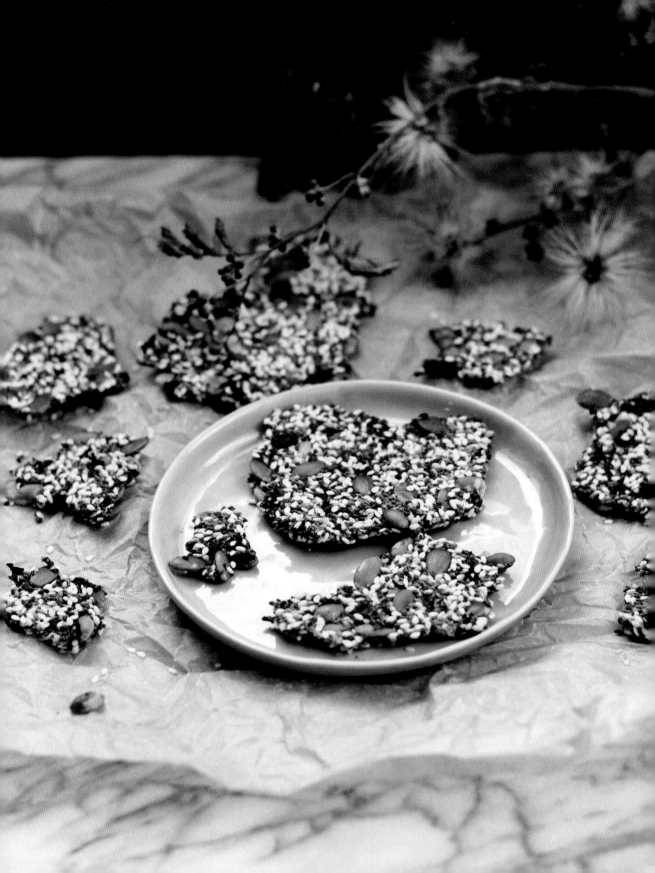

NORI SEED CRACKERS

seaweed, chia seeds, sesame seeds, pumpkin seeds

A cracker without flour, you ask? You've got to bake it to believe it. This is a kind of shortcut cracker recipe because the chia and water are what bind the other ingredients, resulting in a crisp, crunchy cracker. No flour or leavener needed. Now it's pretty much the only cracker we make. Because when a cracker is tasty, healthy, and looks so pretty, why make anything else? We love crumbling ours on top of soups and salads or simply enjoying as is.

MAKES ABOUT 2 DOZEN CRACKERS

½ cup chopped roasted seaweed snack

½ cup chia seeds

½ cup sesame seeds

½ cup pumpkin seeds

¼ teaspoon kosher salt

¼ teaspoon garlic powder (optional)

1. Preheat the oven to 300°F. Line a large baking sheet with parchment paper.

2. Place all the ingredients plus 1 cup of water in a medium-size bowl and give a quick stir to combine. Let rest until the water has been absorbed by the chia, about 2 minutes. The mixture will be wet but should hold its shape when pinched.

3. Dump the mixture onto the prepared baking sheet and spread evenly to a ½- to ¼-inch thickness.

4. Bake for 35 minutes. Remove from the oven, flip the cracker sheet with a spatula, and return the pan to the oven for an additional 30 to 35 minutes, or until the cracker feels hardened and the seeds are toasted but not burned.

5. Remove from the oven and let cool for 5 to 10 minutes. Break up into pieces and enjoy!

HEALING SIPPING BROTH

garlic, ginger, nutritional yeast

Sipping a comforting, soul-nourishing broth is one of life's great pleasures. And during those postpartum months of recovery, it is especially welcome. If you're vegetarian, don't have pounds of bones handy, or don't want to wait eight hours for your broth, we've got you covered. This is a beautiful sipping broth overflowing with deep umami richness from the garlic and nutritional yeast. Yet it's made with a few simple ingredients and develops its flavor in less than an hour. This broth is divine on its own, or you can make it into a meal by adding some soba noodles, sliced scallions, and toasted sesame seeds to the finished broth.

SERVES 4

3 garlic heads

1 (2-inch) knob fresh ginger, peeled and sliced into 5 coins

2 tablespoons olive oil

3 tablespoons nutritional yeast

1½ teaspoons kosher salt

2 tablespoons collagen peptides (optional)

1. Take one garlic head, separate all its cloves, then peel and slightly crush them. Slice off the tops of the remaining two garlic heads and set aside, reserving the tops.

2. In a large stockpot, heat the olive oil over medium heat. Add the crushed garlic and ginger. Cook for 8 to 10 minutes over medium heat, stirring throughout to prevent the garlic from sticking to the pan or burning. The garlic and ginger are done when the garlic is soft and golden brown. Be careful not to burn.

3. Add 7 cups of water and the nutritional yeast, salt, and reserved garlic heads (skin on), along with their tops, to the pot and bring to a boil. Lower the heat and let simmer for 30 minutes, or until the garlic has completely softened.

4. Place a colander or mesh sieve over a bowl. Pour the broth through the colander to strain, leaving a clear, finished broth remaining in the bowl.

5. Enjoy immediately, or bring to room temperature and store in an airtight container in the refrigerator for up to 1 week or in the freezer for up to 1 month. Reheat on the stovetop when ready to enjoy.

6. Optional: For a protein boost, stir 2 tablespoons of collagen peptides into your mug of hot broth.

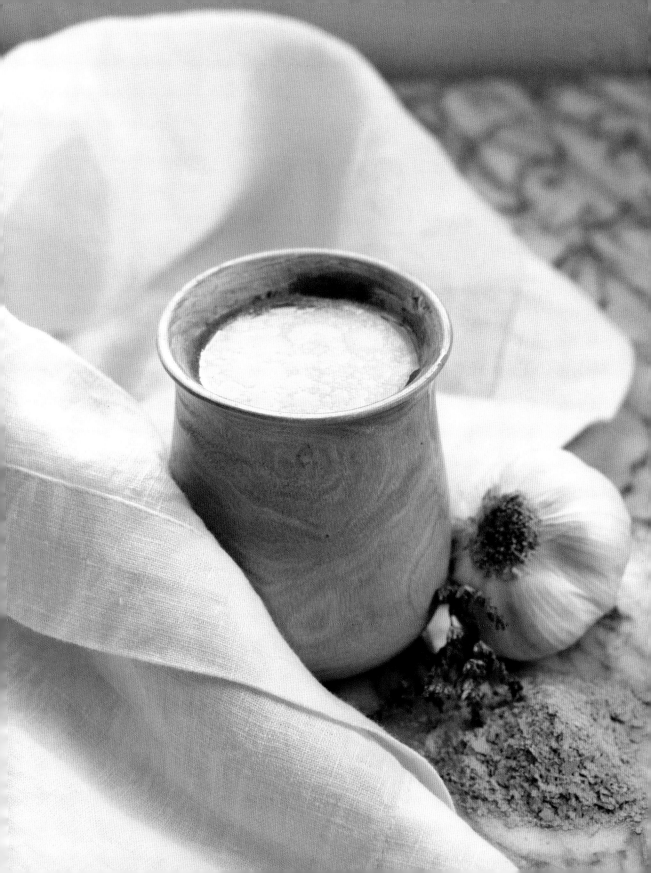

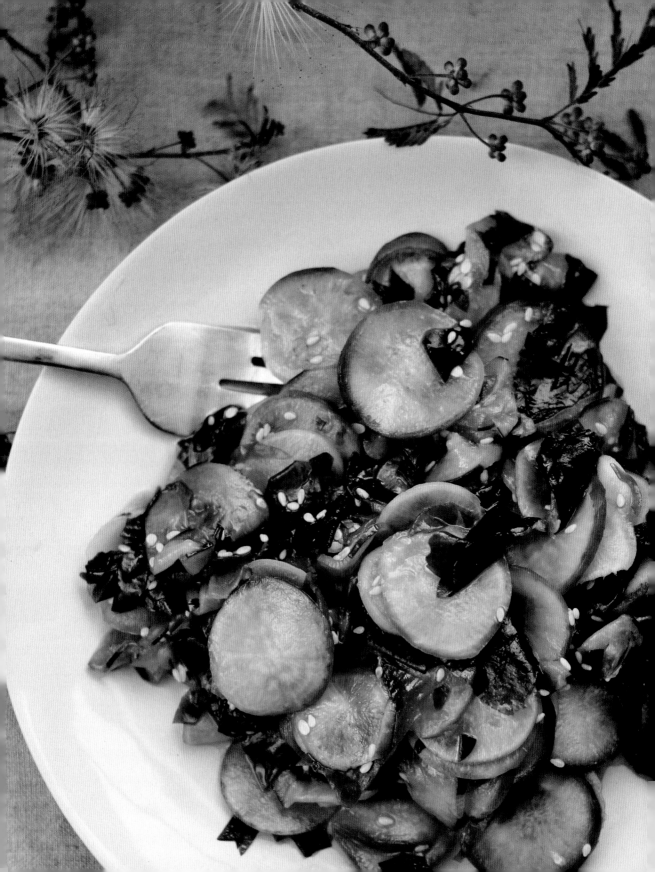

HYDRATING SEAWEED SALAD

seaweed, sesame seeds

If you crave cold seaweed salads from your local Japanese restaurant, but have never tried making one yourself, we're here to help! You can find dried seaweed in the international foods aisle of most major grocery stores and certainly any Asian superstore. This recipe will show you how easy it is to prepare delicious seaweed salads at home. Once you see how simple it is, you'll be hooked. Here is our basic wakame seaweed salad to get you started. There is nothing quite as refreshing on a hot day as a cold seaweed salad with vinegar and cucumber. When your body feels exhausted, this is exactly the snack that will help replenish minerals, hydrate, and invigorate you.

SERVES 2

2 tablespoons dried wakame flakes

2 cups cold water

1 large cucumber, sliced thinly

1 bunch radishes, trimmed and sliced thinly

¼ teaspoon salt

3 tablespoons rice vinegar

2 teaspoons honey

½ teaspoon sesame oil

¼ teaspoon tamari

1½ teaspoons sesame seeds

1. In a small bowl, soak the dried wakame flakes in the cold water until soft, about 10 minutes.

2. Place the cucumber and radish slices in a medium-size bowl and toss with the salt. Let sit until their liquid is leached out, about 5 minutes.

3. Drain the seaweed and squeeze out any additional water. Place in another medium-size bowl. If there are large pieces of seaweed, you may want to cut them up to make them smaller.

4. Drain the cucumbers and radishes and also squeeze out any remaining liquid. Add to the seaweed.

5. In a small bowl, whisk together the rice vinegar, honey, sesame oil, tamari, and sesame seeds, to make a dressing.

6. Pour the dressing over the seaweed and vegetables and toss until evenly coated. Enjoy immediately or cover and refrigerate for later.

KOREAN TACO BITES

millet, seaweed, sesame seeds

Kimchi is a fermented vegetable dish, usually cabbage or radish, originating in South Korea. Not only is it slightly sour, spicy, with a deep, complex flavor profile, it is a probiotic superfood. While breastfeeding, eating probiotic foods can have the added benefit of passing on good bacteria to Baby and helping him or her develop a strong immune system and gut. These little tacos are made by using roasted seaweed snack as the wrapper and filling it with a bit of grains, kimchi, and a sprinkling of sesame seeds. It really is the perfect bite.

MAKES ABOUT 1 DOZEN BITES

½ cup uncooked short-grain white rice

1 tablespoon uncooked millet

1 (0.35-ounce) package roasted seaweed snack

⅓ cup kimchi, chopped

2 tablespoons sesame seeds

1 teaspoon toasted sesame oil (optional)

1. Combine the rice and millet in a colander and rinse thoroughly under running water, until the water runs clear. Cook in a saucepan according to the package directions, or use a rice cooker to cook.

2. When the rice blend is finished cooking, scoop about a tablespoon onto a piece of roasted seaweed snack and top with a heaping teaspoon of kimchi and a sprinkling of sesame seeds. If desired, you can close the taco by spreading a bit of sesame oil on the top of the seaweed snack and sealing the two ends together. Repeat with the remaining cooked rice and seaweed snacks.

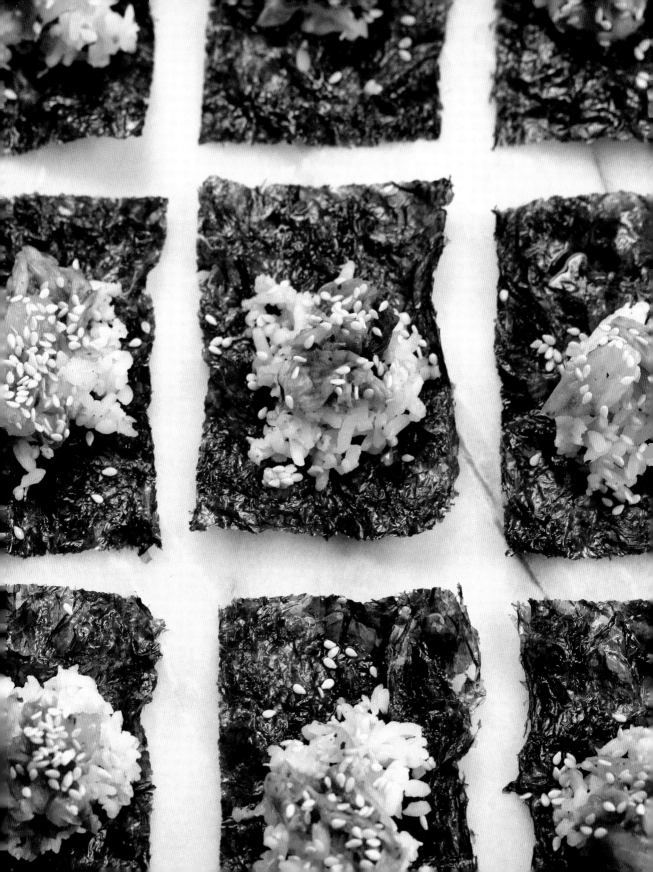

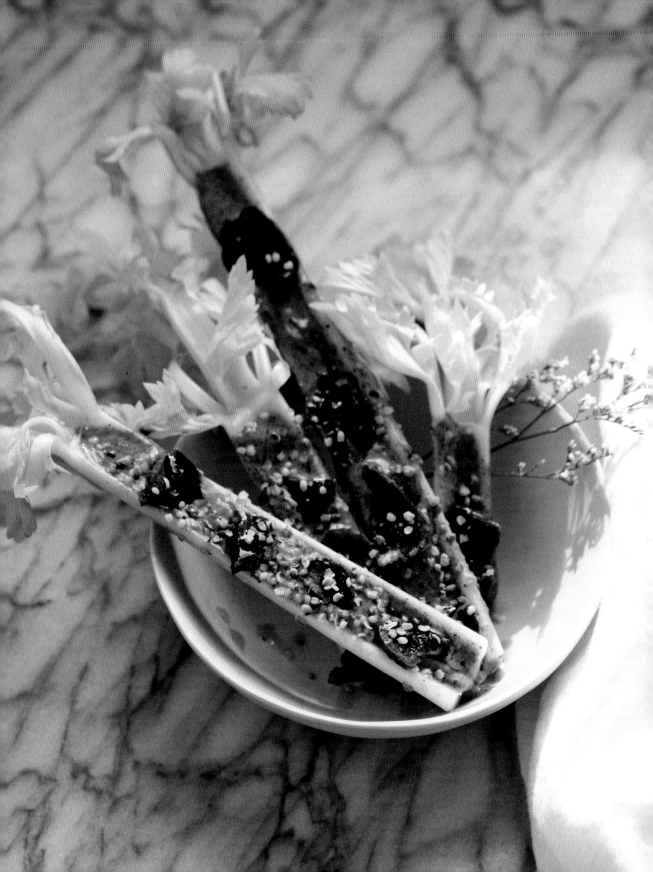

QUEEN ANTS ON A LOG

almond butter, figs, hemp seeds, chia seeds

Ants on a log was a classic snack while we were growing up and brings good memories of lazy summer afternoons. Because it required no cooking, it might have been the first snack you were allowed to prepare by yourself. And maybe like us, you felt pretty fancy about it. Now we are the moms who will be helping to create these food memories for our own children. This version gets an upgrade with the delicious combination of figs and almond butter, and the finishing touches—a drizzle of honey and a sprinkle of crunchy seeds and flaky salt—make it fit for the queen in you. We hope these playful snacks help channel your inner child, bring a smile to your face, and remind you of how the love of food connects us all.

MAKES 8 LOGS (2 TO 4 SERVINGS)

4 celery ribs

¼ cup almond butter

4 dried figs, chopped

1 teaspoon hemp seeds

1 teaspoon chia seeds

1 tablespoon honey

¼ teaspoon sea salt flakes

1. Rinse the celery and cut in half crosswise for a total of eight sticks. Place on a plate with their indentations upward.

2. With a butter knife, fill in the celery sticks with the almond butter, spreading evenly from top to bottom.

3. Arrange the chopped figs along each celery stick and press gently into almond butter.

4. Sprinkle the hemp and chia seeds on top. Finish with a drizzle of honey and a sprinkling of sea salt.

ZOOK ROLL-UPS

carrot, dill, basil

Variety is the spice of life, they say, and that is especially true when it comes to snacking on raw veggies. We've all gotten stuck in a rut of baby carrots and cucumbers. Here is a new way to sneak in some vegetable snacking besides the usual sticks and dips. These roll-ups are brimming with herbs and creamy cheese and raw veggies, but without the usual crunch. Instead, they are soft, fresh, and light, with a salty kick from the goat cheese. A tip to get the cheese to spread on more easily is to pat the zucchini slices dry first before spreading.

MAKES 6 ROLL-UPS

1 medium zucchini

1 medium carrot

3 tablespoons whipped cream cheese

1 teaspoon chopped fresh dill

1 teaspoon chopped fresh chives

1 teaspoon lemon zest

12 fresh basil leaves

1. With a mandoline or vegetable peeler, thinly slice the zucchini into ribbons—long, wide, flat strips. You want the zucchini thin enough to be flexible and pliable but not so thin that it is falling apart. Do the same for the carrot.

2. Lay the zucchini ribbons flat on a cutting board. Apply about ½ teaspoon of goat cheese to a zucchini ribbon and spread an even layer along the ribbon.

3. Top evenly with the carrot strips, dill, chives, lemon zest, and two basil leaves.

4. From one side, pick up the edge and begin to roll it up, zucchini side out, until it is completely rolled and you have a pinwheel. Repeat for the remaining zucchini ribbons. Enjoy immediately.

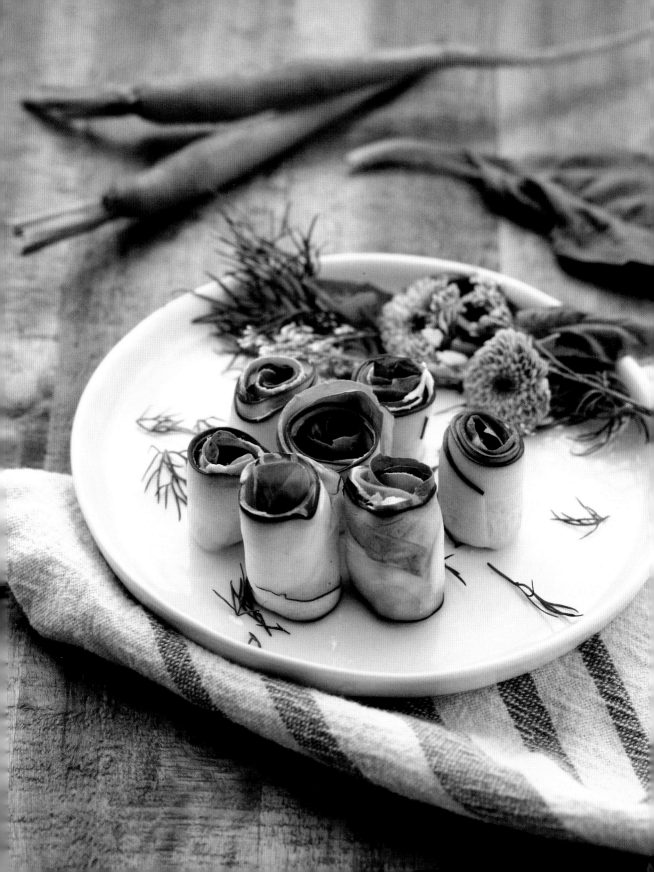

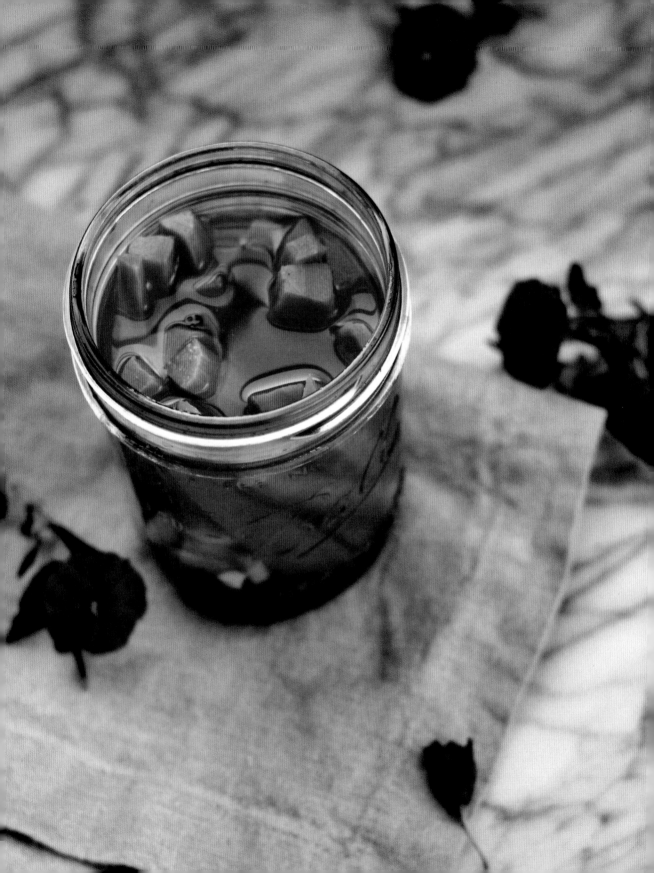

QUICK-PICKLED CARROT STICKS

carrots, cumin, garlic

Some people love to snack on sweets, and others on salty things, and then there are those of us who swear by pickles. If the process of canning seems a little intimidating and you don't want to wait that long, the quick pickle is where it's at. You can use a ton of different vegetables and even change up the brining liquid with all different fun combinations of spices and vinegars. We put together these cumin-kissed, crunchy, garlicky carrot sticks and never looked back. You can feel good about eating the whole jar.

SERVES 2 TO 4

3 medium-size carrots, cut into sticks

½ cup white vinegar

1 tablespoon cumin seeds

4 or 5 garlic cloves, lightly smashed

½ teaspoon kosher salt

¼ teaspoon peppercorns

1. Arrange the carrot sticks upright in a 16-ounce wide-mouth mason jar. Set aside.

2. Combine the vinegar, ½ cup of water, and the cumin seeds, garlic, salt, and peppercorns in a small saucepan and heat until just boiling.

3. Pour the hot mixture over the carrots. Let cool.

4. When completely cooled, top the jar with its lid and refrigerate. Enjoy cold. The pickles will keep for about 2 weeks in the fridge.

VEGGIE DILL DIP

Greek-style yogurt, fresh dill

Maybe it's the mom in us or maybe it's the toddler in us, but sometimes we could all use some help eating our fresh veggies, are we right? This creamy dip will make you keep going in for more, and before you know it, you've polished off a plate of vitamins and minerals. Keep some handy for anytime those munchies strike.

SERVES 4

1 cup Greek-style yogurt

2 tablespoons fresh dill, chopped

½ teaspoon garlic powder

½ teaspoon onion powder

½ teaspoon Himalayan pink salt

Mix all the ingredients together until smooth. Refrigerate until cool, 1 to 2 hours. Serve chilled with an assortment of fresh veggies.

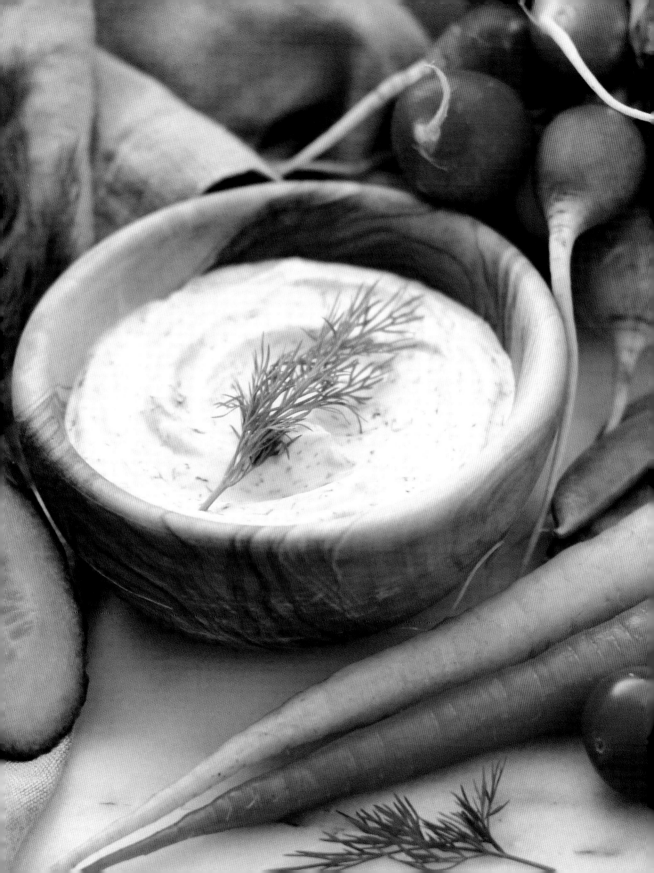

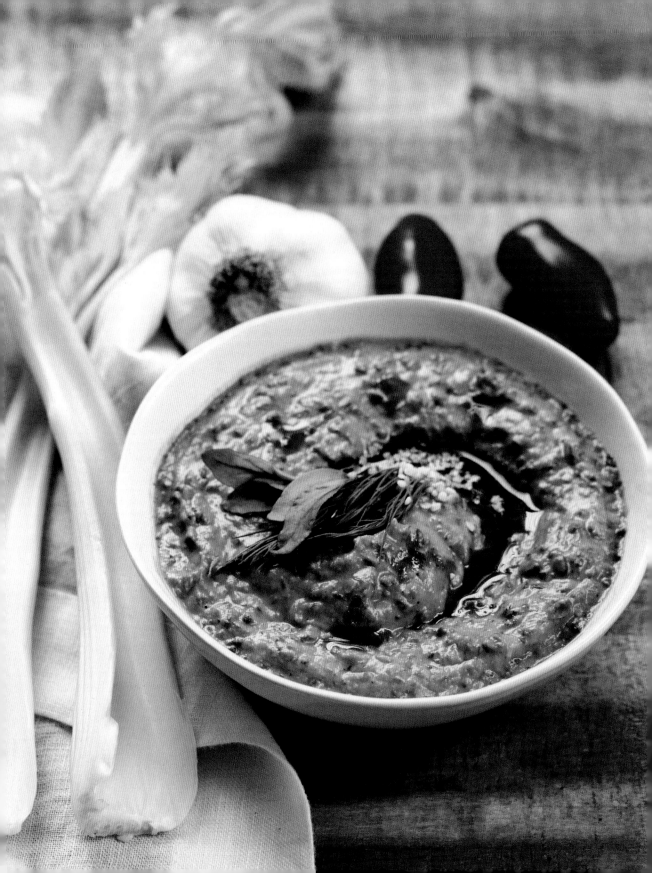

ROASTED GARLIC LENTIL DIP

garlic, lentils, nutritional yeast, cumin

One of our favorite aromas in the kitchen is the scent of roasting garlic. This is a deeply satisfying dip with complex flavors that continue to develop after a few days in the fridge. You can use it as a spread on toast, a dip with pita chips or veggie sticks, or as part of a meze platter with olives and roasted vegetables and cheeses.

SERVES 2

1 garlic head

2 tablespoons extra-virgin olive oil

1 (15-ounce) can lentils, drained and rinsed

1 tablespoon freshly squeezed lemon juice

1½ teaspoons nutritional yeast

½ teaspoon ground cumin

½ teaspoon kosher salt

¼ teaspoon smoked paprika

1. Preheat the oven to 400°F.

2. Cut off and discard the top of the garlic head so the cloves are exposed. Drizzle 1 tablespoon of the olive oil on top of the garlic. Place on a rimmed baking sheet. Bake the garlic for 30 to 35 minutes, or until the cloves are deeply golden and soft when pinched.

3. Squeeze out the roasted garlic cloves from the skin and place in a food processor along with the remaining ingredients, including the reserved tablespoon of oil.

4. Pulse until smooth. Serve immediately and refrigerate any leftovers. Will keep for 2 to 3 days.

PEANUT BUTTER POWER POPCORN

coconut oil, peanut butter, flaxseeds

A whole-grain snack that is full of fiber, popcorn has gotten a bad rap as junk food. Prepared from scratch on the stovetop, without all the salt and artificial butter, popcorn is actually a very wholesome snack that delivers an impressive dose of antioxidants and can even aid in digestion. We thought we'd improve on popcorn's benefits by upping the protein content, and flavor, with a coating of creamy peanut butter, coconut sugar, and flax. So, kick up your feet, and enjoy your nighttime pumping session with a movie and a big bowl of power popcorn.

SERVES 4

2½ teaspoons coconut oil

⅓ cup unpopped popcorn kernels

3 tablespoons natural creamy peanut
butter

2 teaspoons coconut sugar

⅛ to ¼ teaspoon salt, or to taste

1 tablespoon ground flaxseeds

1. Heat ½ teaspoon of the coconut oil over medium-high heat in a medium-size saucepan with a lid. When the oil is heated through, add the popcorn kernels.

2. Swirl the kernels in the oil, watching closely, just until they begin to pop, then quickly cover with a lid. Lightly shake the covered pot back and forth over the heat.

3. When the popping has slowed to one pop every few seconds, pour the popcorn into a large bowl and set aside.

4. In the same saucepan, combine the remaining 2 teaspoons of coconut oil with the peanut butter and coconut sugar and heat the mixture over low heat, stirring gently, for about 30 seconds, or until melted and well blended.

5. Pour the warm peanut butter mixture over the popcorn and mix until the popcorn is evenly coated.

6. Sprinkle with the salt and ground flax to taste and mix to evenly distribute.

7. Enjoy warm, or place it in the freezer for a few minutes to dry and cool before serving.

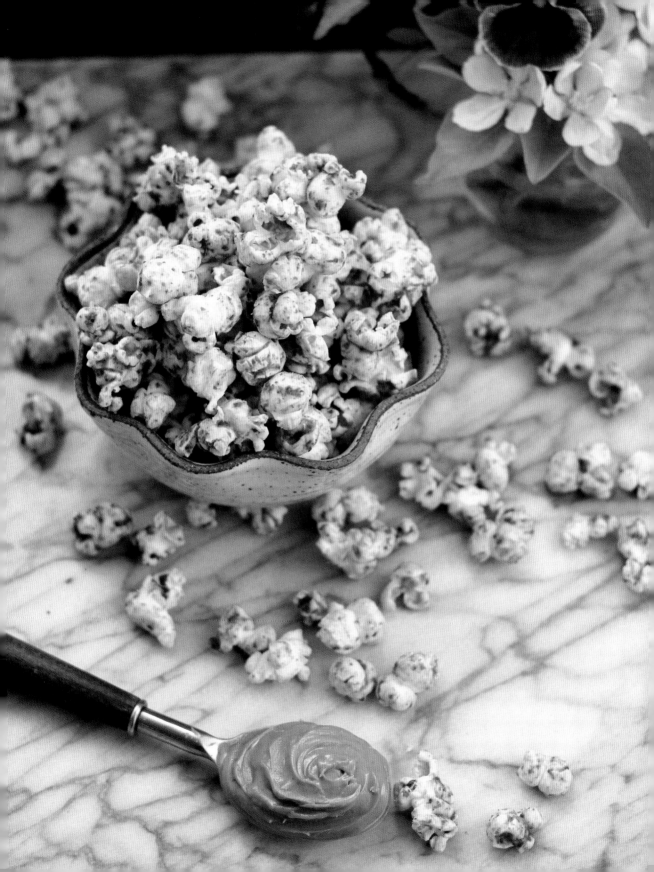

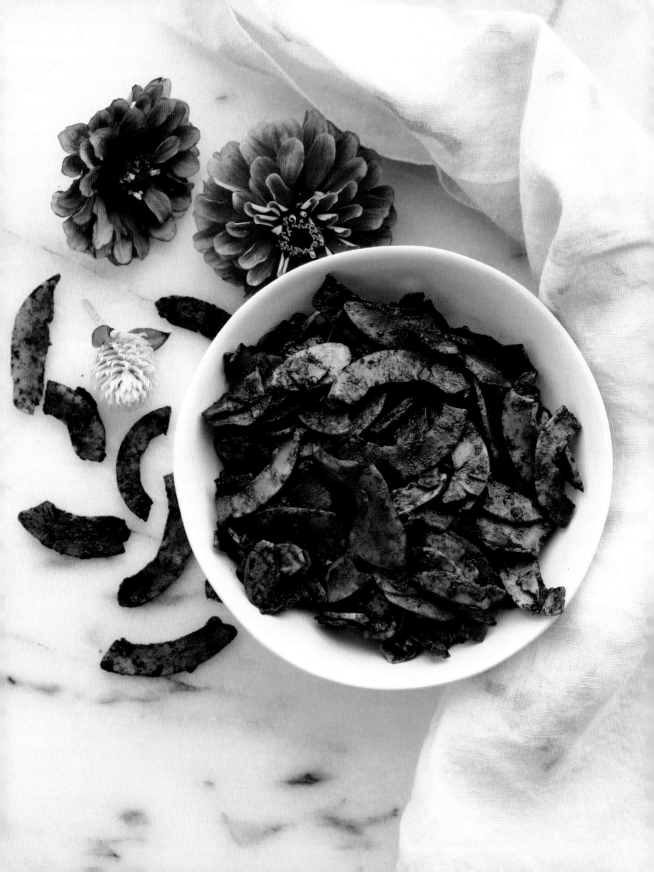

TOASTED COCOA-NUT CHIPS

coconut, almonds, nutritional yeast

When coconut flakes are baked, they develop an irresistible crunch. If you like crispy, chocolaty, salty, nutty snacks (yes please!), you're going to love these "chips." When we make these, the adults and kids gobble them up at such record speed, the pan has barely cooled before they are gone. They are that good. You can eat these straight up or sprinkle them on top of vanilla yogurt or a smoothie.

MAKES ABOUT 2 CUPS CHIPS

2 cups unsweetened dried coconut (large flakes)

½ cup raw sliced almonds

2 tablespoons extra-virgin coconut oil

¼ cup pure maple syrup

3 tablespoons unsweetened cocoa powder

1 tablespoon nutritional yeast

¼ teaspoon salt

1. Preheat the oven to 325°F.

2. In a medium-size bowl, combine the coconut and almonds. Set aside.

3. In a small saucepan over low heat, whisk together the coconut oil, maple syrup, cocoa powder, nutritional yeast, and salt and heat for about 2 minutes, or until warmed.

4. Pour the warmed sauce over the coconut mixture, mixing until it's evenly coated. Fold gently to avoid breaking up the coconut. You want to keep the flakes in big pieces.

5. Pour the coconut mixture onto an ungreased baking sheet and spread out evenly.

6. Bake for 5 minutes, give the mixture a good stir, then bake for another 10 minutes, stirring at the 5-minute point, until the coconut is fragrant and about half of the sauce has baked off. Be careful not to burn.

7. Remove from the oven and allow the chips to cool for 10 minutes. The chips will get crunchier as they cool. Store at room temperature in an airtight container for up to 2 weeks.

Dinner

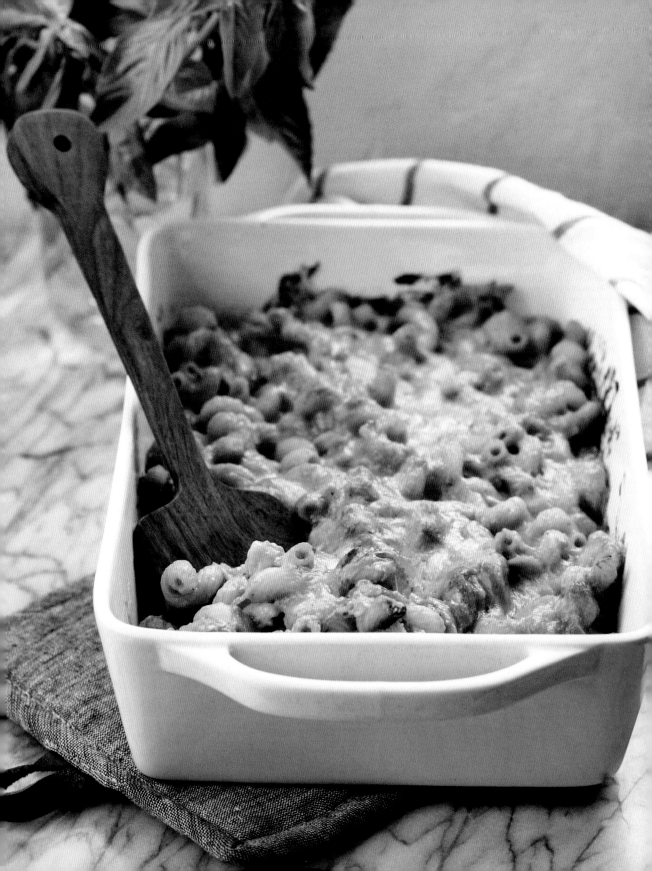

BUTTERNUT SQUASH MAC AND CHEESE
with NUTRITIONAL YEAST

chickpeas, nutritional yeast, butternut squash

If you're pregnant and looking to pack your freezer full of easy, reheatable meals that will please the whole family, start with this recipe. When Baby comes home, you'll want to spend all the time you can getting acquainted with each other. You'll most likely be exhausted, overwhelmed, even in a daze of sorts. It's best to have some of those first weeks of meals sorted out and ready, so you're not left scrambling to order takeout every night. This makes a ton and can feed a crowd, so if freezing first, feel free to split it up into a few smaller meals.

SERVES 8 TO 10

- 2 cups uncooked chickpea pasta shells or spirals
- 3 cups uncooked pasta shells or spirals
- 1 tablespoon olive oil
- 1 medium-size onion, sliced thinly
- 4 tablespoons (½ stick, 2 ounces) unsalted grass-fed butter
- 1 tablespoon all-purpose flour
- 2 cups whole milk

- ½ teaspoon ground mustard
- ¼ cup nutritional yeast
- ¼ teaspoon ground nutmeg
- ¼ teaspoon garlic powder
- 1 teaspoon Himalayan pink salt
- ½ teaspoon freshly ground black pepper
- 1½ cups or 1 (15-ounce) can butternut squash puree
- 2 cups shredded sharp Cheddar cheese

1. Cook the pastas according to their package directions. Drain and rinse. Set aside in one of the pots used to cook the pasta.

2. Heat the olive oil in a skillet over medium-low heat. Add the onion and cook, stirring occasionally, until golden brown and caramelized, 20 to 25 minutes. Add to the drained pasta and stir to incorporate, then cover with a lid and set aside while you prepare the remaining ingredients.

3. Meanwhile, preheat the oven to 375°F.

4. In a large saucepan over medium-low heat, melt the butter. Whisk in the flour and stir for about 2 minutes. Whisk in the milk, ground mustard, nutritional yeast,

continued on page 114

nutmeg, garlic powder, salt, and pepper and stir until the sauce has thickened. Whisk in the butternut squash puree until smooth. Stir in 1 cup of the cheese until melted, then remove from the heat.

5. Add the pasta mixture to the sauce and stir until well combined.

6. Pour into a 9 by 13-inch baking pan and top with the remaining cup of cheese.

7. Bake for 30 to 35 minutes, or until hot throughout and bubbly around the edges. Serve warm.

Variation: Add 2 cups of wilted spinach or kale to the pasta in step 5 and then mix with the sauce.

CHANA MASALA–STUFFED SWEET POTATOES

sweet potatoes, garlic, cumin, chickpeas

If you like twice-baked potatoes, here is an extremely flavorful take on them without the white potatoes and heaps of cheese. In this version, we use sweet potatoes, and ours are stuffed with lactogenic spices and chickpeas (these legumes are chana *in Hindi). The roasting method slightly caramelizes the outer edges of the potatoes, creating irresistible sweet, crunchy corners. We last served these for a dinner party and they flew off the platter, followed by lots of recipe requests. Serve these sweet potatoes alongside a side of jasmine rice spiked with cumin seeds and some lemony yogurt and you'll be one happy mama.*

SERVES 6

3 medium-size to large sweet potatoes

3 tablespoons olive or sunflower oil

Himalayan pink salt

1 medium-size onion, diced finely

2 garlic cloves, minced

1 (½-inch) piece fresh ginger, peeled and minced

1 medium-size tomato, diced

1 teaspoon garam masala

1 teaspoon ground turmeric

½ teaspoon ground coriander

½ teaspoon cumin seeds

½ teaspoon ground cumin

1 (14-ounce) can chickpeas, drained and rinsed

Juice of ½ lemon

Thinly sliced scallions, for garnish

Fresh cilantro, for garnish

1. Preheat the oven to 400°F.

2. Slice the sweet potatoes in half lengthwise and drizzle with 2 tablespoons of the oil. Rub the halves together to help evenly coat them with oil, then top with a light sprinkle of pink salt. Lay the sweet potato halves, cut side down, on an ungreased baking sheet and bake for 25 to 30 minutes, or until tender when poked with a fork. Remove from the oven and set aside to cool.

3. Heat the remaining tablespoon of oil in a medium-size saucepan over medium-high heat. Add the onion and cook until translucent and lightly browned, about 5 minutes. Stir in the garlic, ginger, tomato, garam masala, turmeric, coriander, cumin seeds, ground cumin, and ½ teaspoon of the pink salt and cook for 3 to 5 minutes, until nice and fragrant.

continued on page 117

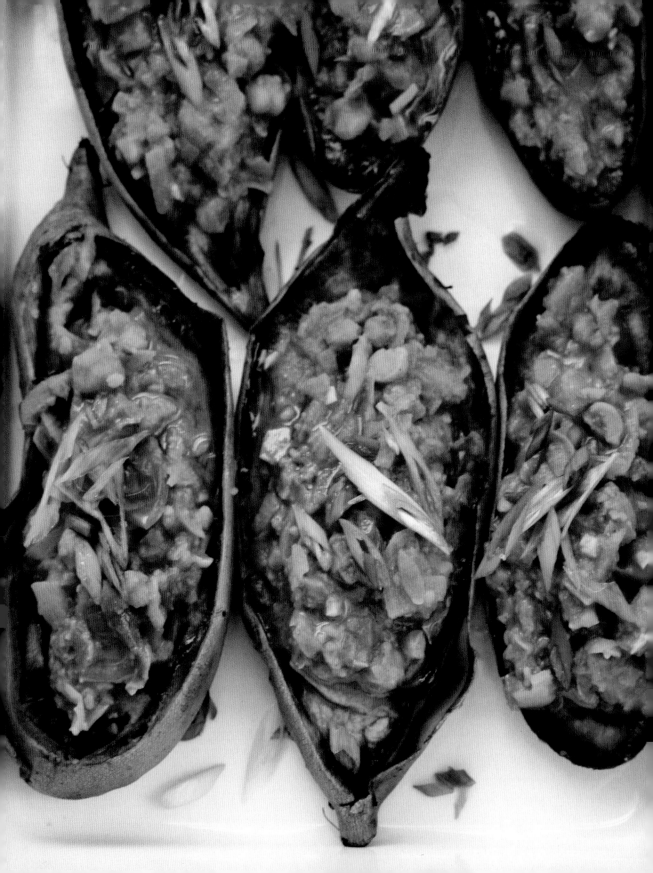

4. Stir in the chickpeas, 1 cup of water, and the lemon juice. Using a potato masher, gently crush some of the chickpeas, leaving some whole. Cover the pan with a lid, reduce heat to low, and cook for 10 minutes.

5. While the chana masala cooks, begin scooping the sweet potato flesh from the skin to make six "boats," leaving a ½-inch perimeter of sweet potato around the skin.

6. Take half of the scooped-out sweet potato and give it a rough chop, and then stir it into the pot of chana masala. Set aside remaining sweet potato for another dish or for baby food.

7. Fill the sweet potato boats with a heaping serving of chana masala. Bake for 5 minutes to heat through.

8. Top with scallions and cilantro. Serve immediately.

QUINOA AND ROASTED TOMATOES AND GARLIC with LEMON CUMIN DRESSING

garlic, quinoa, cumin, lentils

Don't let the intimidating list of ingredients scare you off from this recipe. This one actually comes together in under thirty minutes. The tomatoes and garlic are roasting while the quinoa cooks, and the dressing takes just a minute to throw together in a food processor. It will look as though you spent hours on it, and is brimming with healthy fats and a big kick of protein from the quinoa. You will truly look and feel like a supermom with this meal, which is ideal for potlucks, get-togethers, or simply a tasty weeknight dinner.

SERVES 6

1 pint cherry tomatoes

15 to 20 garlic cloves

1 tablespoon extra-virgin olive oil

¼ teaspoon salt

Freshly ground black pepper

1 cup uncooked quinoa

3 cups vegetable stock

LEMON CUMIN DRESSING:

Juice of ½ lemon (about
  1 tablespoon)

¼ cup extra-virgin olive oil

¼ teaspoon salt

½ teaspoon ground cumin

TO ASSEMBLE:

1 (12-ounce) jar marinated
  artichokes, drained

½ cup pitted kalamata olives

2 teaspoons cumin seeds

1 (15-ounce) can black lentils,
  drained and rinsed

1. Preheat the oven to 400°F.

2. Cut the cherry tomatoes in half and lightly smash each garlic clove with the side of a chef's knife. Place both on a rimmed baking sheet. Top with the olive oil, salt, and a few grinds of pepper. Toss together until the tomatoes and garlic are well coated.

3. Roast for 20 minutes, stirring halfway through, or until the tomatoes and garlic are soft and caramelized. Set aside.

continued on page 120

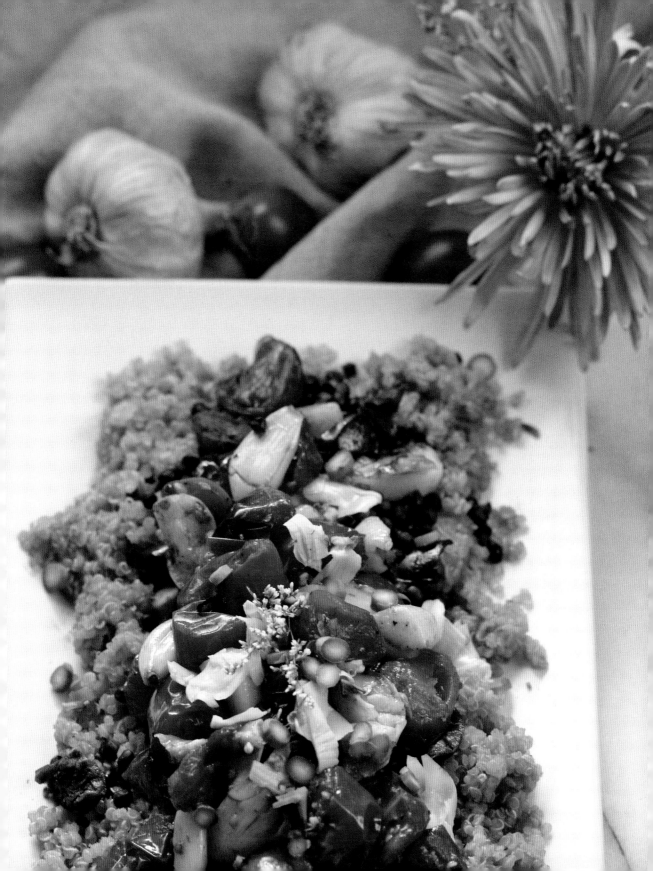

4. Meanwhile, rinse the quinoa in a fine sieve until the water runs clear. Place in a small, dry saucepan over medium heat. Toast the quinoa for 2 to 3 minutes, stirring once or twice. Add the vegetable stock, increase the heat to medium-high, and bring to a boil.

5. Cover and lower the heat to low. Let the quinoa simmer for 10 to 15 minutes, or until the liquid is absorbed, then turn off the heat and let sit for another 5 minutes. Uncover and fluff the quinoa with fork.

6. Prepare the dressing: Combine the lemon juice, olive oil, salt, and cumin in a small bowl and whisk together.

7. Roughly chop the artichokes and olives. Place the cumin seeds in a dry saucepan over medium heat and toast for 3 to 4 minutes, or until fragrant. Remove from the pan.

8. To assemble the salad, place the quinoa on a large serving platter and drizzle with one third of the dressing. Top with the lentils and drizzle with another third of the dressing, then add the olives, artichokes, and roasted tomatoes and garlic. Top with the toasted cumin seeds. If desired, drizzle the remaining dressing or set aside for future use.

FAJITA-STUFFED PEPPERS

garlic, cumin, bulgur

Here is a new twist on your classic stuffed pepper for a simple weeknight meal. Instead of white rice and ground beef, we use bulgur and black beans. The stuffing is generously seasoned with a blend of smoky, savory spices, and together with the slightly sweet roasted bell pepper, makes a very satisfying and comforting meal. These peppers are highly customizable. Brown rice or quinoa would work in place of the bulgur, and chickpeas or pinto beans could replace the black beans.

SERVES 4

1 tablespoon chili powder

1½ teaspoons smoked paprika

½ teaspoon onion powder

¼ teaspoon garlic powder

¼ teaspoon ground cumin

½ teaspoon salt

1 teaspoon dark brown sugar

3 tablespoons olive oil

½ large yellow onion, chopped finely

3 garlic cloves, minced

2 cups cooked bulgur

1 (15-ounce) can black beans, drained and rinsed

4 large bell peppers

Optional garnishes: Queso fresco and chopped cilantro

1. Preheat the oven to 350°F.

2. Place all the spices, salt, and brown sugar in a small bowl along with 2 tablespoons of the olive oil. Mix to combine and set aside.

3. Heat the remaining tablespoon of olive oil in a large skillet over medium-high heat. Add the onion and cook until softened and translucent, 4 to 5 minutes. Add the garlic and cook until fragrant, about 30 seconds more.

4. Add the bulgur, black beans, and the spiced oil and continue to cook until everything is heated through and well coated, 2 to 3 minutes. Remove from the heat.

5. Cut the tops off the bell peppers and carefully remove and discard the seeds and membranes, trying not to pierce the sides of the peppers. Place the prepared peppers upright in a 9-inch square baking dish. If necessary, trim the bottom of the peppers to help them stand up properly.

continued on page 122

6. Using a spoon, evenly fill each hollowed-out pepper with about ¾ cup of the bulgur mixture.

7. Cover the stuffed peppers with foil. Carefully transfer the baking dish to the oven and bake for about 1 hour, or until the peppers are tender and can be pierced with a fork. Serve immediately.

Variation: Add 1 pound of boneless, skinless chicken thighs, cut into 1-inch cubes, to the onion in step 3 and cook until cooked through.

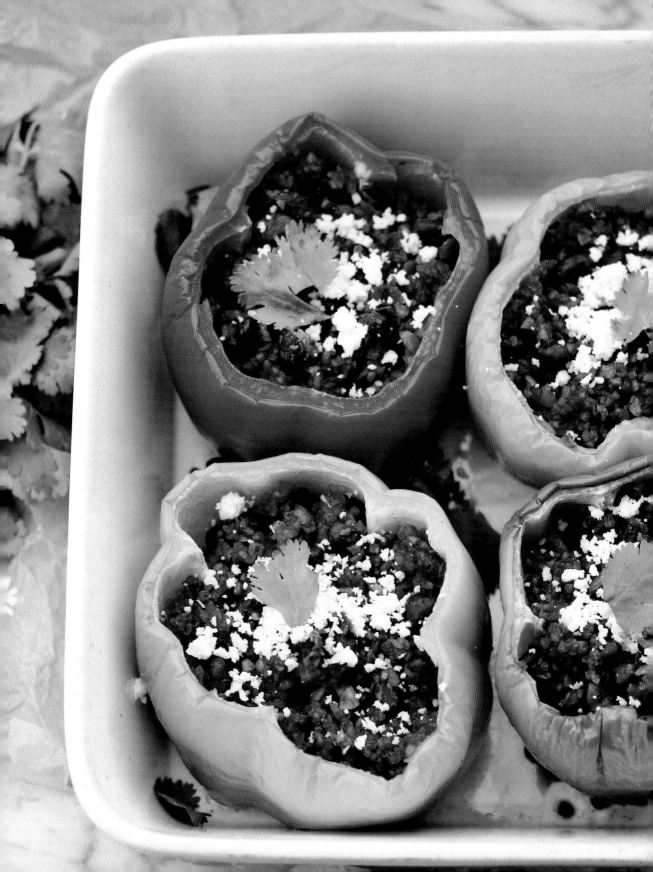

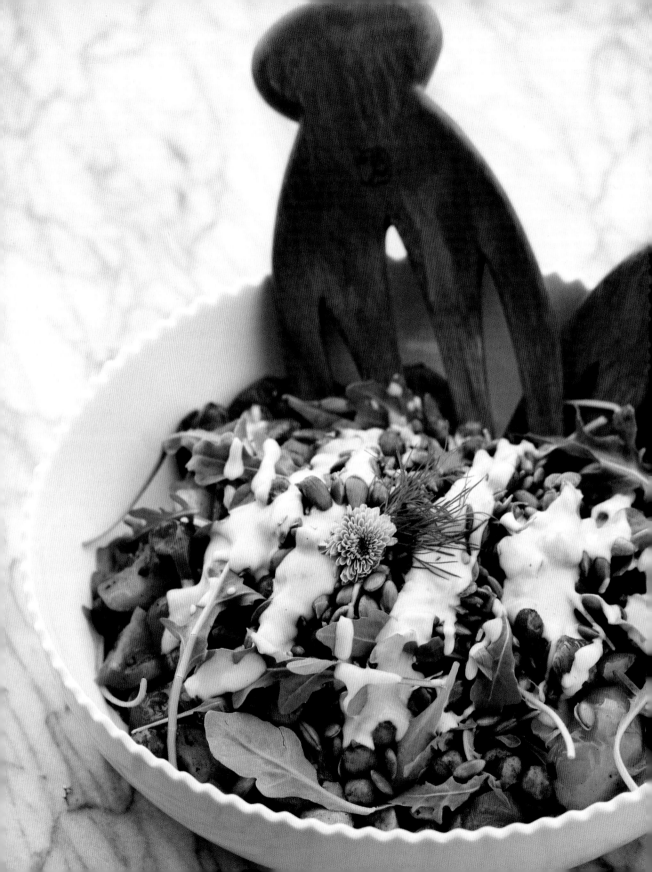

ROASTED SUMMER VEGETABLES with GARLIC TAHINI SAUCE

 garlic, chickpeas, cumin, pumpkin seeds

Cold, crisp salads have their place at the table, without a doubt, but have you tried making a salad with roasted vegetables instead of raw? It's a game-changer. Yes, this is a long list of ingredients, but the dish itself is not difficult or time-consuming to prepare, and the result is so worth it. We promise. Cooking the vegetables in a single layer encourages caramelization and brings out their natural sweetness. This dish presents beautifully and is ideal for feeding a large group or entertaining. All the elements travel well and can be enjoyed warm or cold, so you can feel good about taking this dish to a potluck or making any of the components ahead of time.

SERVES 6

GARLIC TAHINI SAUCE:

⅓ cup tahini

2 garlic cloves, crushed and minced into a paste

3 tablespoons freshly squeezed lemon juice

1 teaspoon salt

2 tablespoons extra-virgin olive oil

CHICKPEAS:

1 (15-ounce) can chickpeas, drained and rinsed

1½ tablespoons extra-virgin olive oil

½ teaspoon salt

1 teaspoon ground turmeric

1 teaspoon ground cumin

SUMMER VEGETABLES:

¼ cup extra-virgin olive oil

2 small zucchini, peeled and chopped into 1- to 1½-inch pieces

1 yellow squash, peeled and chopped into 1- to 1½-inch pieces

1 large red bell pepper, seeded and stemmed, chopped into 1- to 1½-inch pieces

1 large orange bell pepper, seeded and stemmed, chopped into 1- to 1½-inch pieces

1 pint cherry tomatoes

20 garlic cloves (about 1 head)

½ red onion, chopped roughly

Salt and freshly ground black pepper

1 cup raw pumpkin seeds

2 handfuls baby arugula

continued on page 126

1. Prepare the garlic tahini sauce: Combine all the sauce ingredients plus 3 tablespoons of water in a blender and blend until smooth. Scrape into a small bowl and set aside.

2. Prepare the chickpeas: Preheat the oven to 450°F.

3. In a small bowl, combine the chickpeas, olive oil, salt, turmeric, and cumin and gently stir until well coated.

4. Spread the chickpeas in a single layer on a cookie sheet or roasting pan. Roast in the oven, periodically shaking the cookie sheet to release any steam, until the chickpeas are brown and fragrant, 10 to 12 minutes. Remove from the oven and set aside.

5. Prepare the vegetables: Move the oven rack to the top third of the oven. In a large bowl, combine the olive oil, all the vegetables, and salt and pepper to taste. Spread in a single layer on a cookie sheet. Roast on the top third of the oven until cooked through and the edges have started to brown, 45 to 50 minutes, stirring occasionally to make sure the vegetables do not stick.

6. While the vegetables roast, toast the pumpkin seeds in a large, dry sauté pan over medium heat until they have begun to release their oil, are fragrant, and are just starting to brown, 4 to 5 minutes.

7. Remove the roasted veggies from the oven and return them to their large bowl. Mix in the toasted pumpkin seeds and chickpeas and spread onto a large serving platter. Top with the arugula and drizzle with half of the garlic tahini sauce. Serve hot or at room temperature with the remaining sauce on the side.

Variation: Try replacing the summer squash and tomatoes with autumn and winter veggies, such as sweet potatoes, pumpkin, or butternut squash. Replace the pumpkin seeds with toasted pine nuts.

PASTA with CARROT TOMATO SAUCE

carrots, beet, garlic

For many of us moms, the struggle to work extra vegetables into kid-approved meals is an ongoing challenge. This pasta dish will make both mom and baby happy. The carrots create a velvety texture, and the sweetness of the beets balances the tomatoes' acidity. The result is a delicious, silky-smooth sauce with a gorgeous bright orange hue. We recommend pasta shapes that can grab all of the nutritious sauce, so bowties, penne, and rigatoni are wonderful choices. Also, because we suspect this dish will make lots of appearances on the table over the years, we've added three different variations to change it up a bit.

SERVES 4

CARROT TOMATO SAUCE:

3 tablespoons extra-virgin olive oil

1 yellow onion, diced

2 large carrots, diced (about 2 cups)

1 medium-size golden beet, peeled and diced (about 1 cup)

3 garlic cloves, minced

1 (28-ounce) can peeled tomatoes

1 teaspoon salt

12 ounces bowtie pasta

Toasted pumpkin seeds (see page 126 for how to toast), for garnish

Parmesan cheese, sliced into curls, for garnish (optional)

1. Prepare the sauce: In a large saucepan, warm the oil over medium heat. Add the onion, carrots, and beet and sauté until the onion is slightly translucent, 4 to 5 minutes.

2. Add the garlic, peeled tomatoes with juice, and salt and increase the heat to medium-high. Bring the sauce to a slight boil. Cover with a lid, lower the heat to low, and let the sauce simmer for 1 hour, or until the vegetables are soft.

3. Transfer the cooked sauce to a blender and puree until completely smooth (you may need to do this in batches, depending on the size of your blender). Set aside.

4. Meanwhile, as the sauce is cooking, bring a large pot of lightly salted water to a boil. Add the pasta and cook according to the package directions. When the pasta is done, drain well and return it to the pot.

continued on page 129

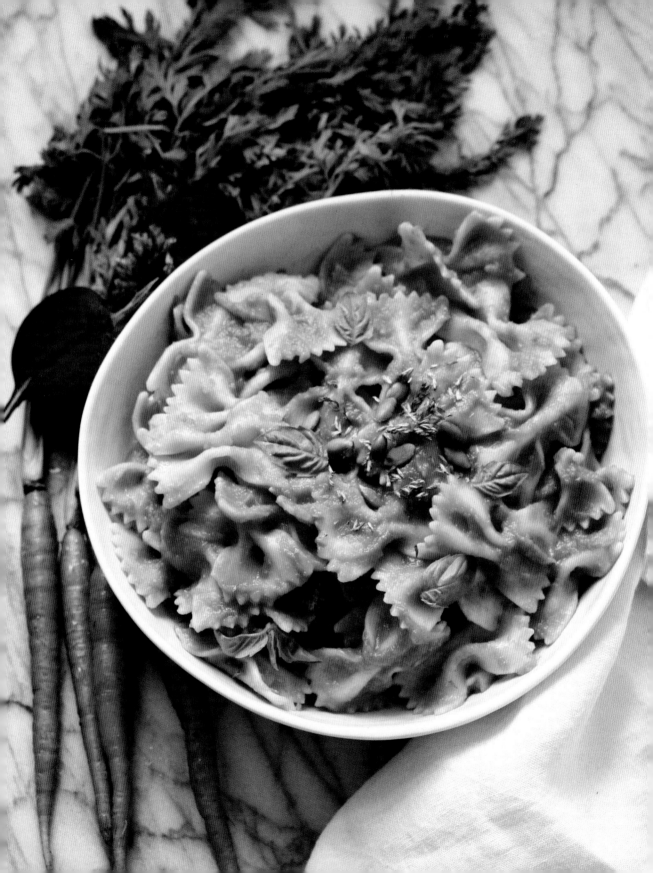

5. Pour the sauce over the cooked pasta and stir to combine. Divide among bowls and serve with a garnish of toasted pumpkin seeds and Parmesan cheese curls. Enjoy immediately.

VARIATIONS:

Bolognese: Stir in 1 pound of cooked ground beef or turkey to the sauce after step 3.

Arrabiata: Add ½ teaspoon of crushed red pepper flakes with the garlic and tomatoes in step 2.

Herb: In the last 5 minutes of cooking time in step 2, add ⅓ cup of fresh basil leaves.

Creamy: After step 3, stir ¼ cup of heavy cream into the sauce until combined.

ROASTED CHICKEN with FENNEL

fennel, garlic, dill

Hurray for one-pan meals when you've got a hungry or sleeping or crying baby on your hip. This meal is everything you want from a dinner: no fuss, no dishes, lots of flavor. This dish really packs a lactation punch from all the fennel and garlic. It may seem like a shocking amount of garlic, but when slowly cooked, garlic really loses its sharp edge and mellows out to flavor this whole dish. If fennel is not readily available, collard greens or kale stands in very nicely. Serve alongside a loaf of crusty rye or sourdough bread to sop up the delicious pan juices.

SERVES 4

4 chicken thighs, bone in and skin on

1 tablespoon plus ½ teaspoon salt

2 tablespoons extra-virgin olive oil

2 fennel bulbs, sliced

1 lemon, sliced, skin on

15 garlic cloves, smashed (from about 1 head)

1 (15.5-ounce) can cannellini beans, drained and rinsed

1 tablespoon fresh dill

Freshly ground black pepper

1. Preheat the oven to 450°F.

2. Pat the chicken breasts dry and sprinkle both sides with 1 tablespoon of the salt.

3. In a medium-size skillet over medium-high heat, heat 1 tablespoon of the oil. When the oil is sizzling, add the chicken thighs, skin down. Sear until the skin is browned and crispy, 4 to 5 minutes. Set aside.

4. In a medium-size bowl, gently toss the fennel, lemon slices, garlic, beans, and dill with remaining tablespoon of olive oil and remaining ½ teaspoon of salt.

5. Transfer the vegetables to a 9 x 12-inch baking dish, spreading to make an even layer. Top with seared chicken thighs.

6. Roast for 30 to 35 minutes, or until the vegetables are caramelized and the chicken is cooked through with its juices running clear. Top with freshly ground pepper. Serve immediately.

Note: Because the lemon in this recipe is used, rind and all, we recommend choosing an organic lemon. Be sure to wash it well before using.

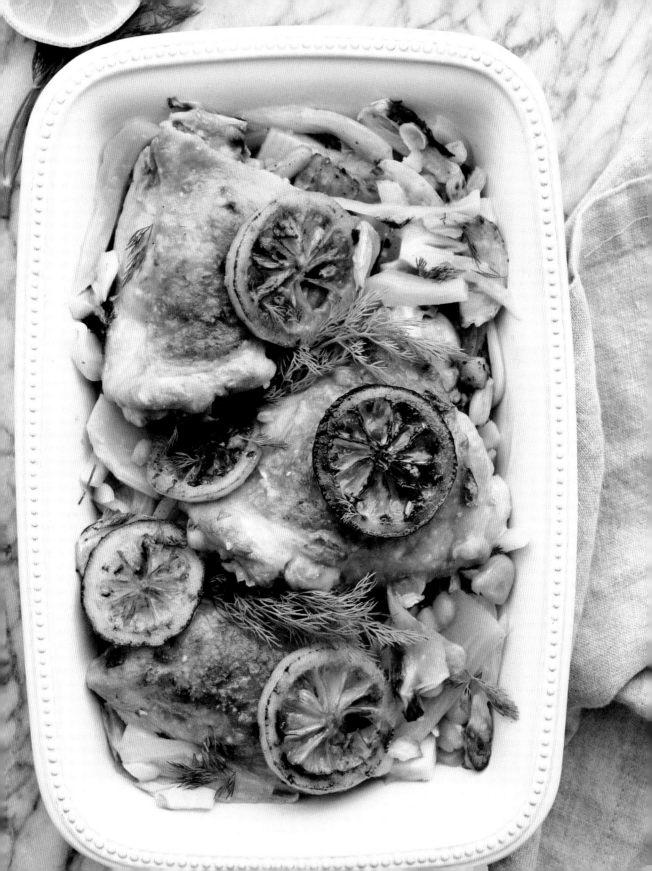

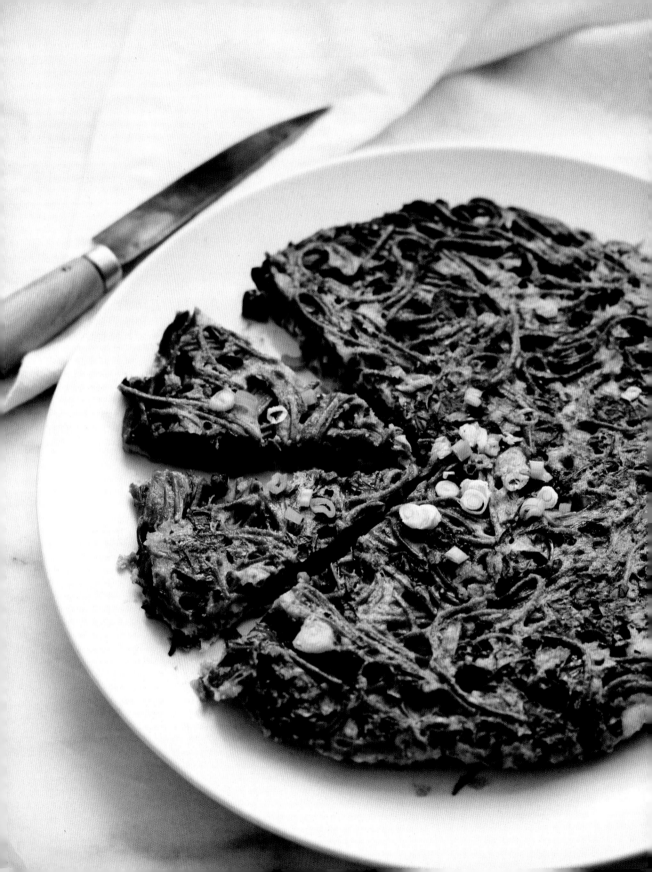

SOBA AND KALE OMELET

soba noodles, kale

Ever heard of spaghetti pie? When there was leftover spaghetti, this tasty curiosity of spaghetti, cheese, and eggs would find its way to our childhood dinner table. All of us loved it, of course. While there isn't much nutritional merit to the original, here is a reinvented version that's packed with lightly sautéed greens and soba noodles. Slice as you would a frittata and serve alongside a cup of miso soup or our Hydrating Seaweed Salad (page 93).

SERVES 4

4 ounces soba noodles

1 teaspoon olive oil

7 lacinato kale leaves, stemmed and cut into ribbons

3 green onions

4 large eggs

¼ cup grated Parmesan cheese

¼ teaspoon garlic powder

½ teaspoon salt

2 tablespoons unsalted grass-fed butter

1. Bring a large pot of water to a boil. Add the soba noodles and cook according to the package directions. When the noodles are done, drain and rinse them thoroughly under cold water until they have cooled. Set aside.

2. Place a 9-inch cast-iron skillet over medium heat and heat the olive oil. Add the kale and green onions. Sauté for 2 to 3 minutes, or until the kale is bright green and slightly wilted. Remove from the pan and set aside.

3. In a medium-size bowl, whisk together the eggs, cheese, garlic powder, and salt. Add the cooled soba noodles and the kale mixture and stir until everything is coated with egg.

4. In the same skillet as used for the kale, melt 1 tablespoon of the butter over low heat. Pour in the egg mixture. Cook over low heat until the eggs begin to set on the bottom but are still slightly wet on top, about 10 minutes. You should be able to use a spatula to gently lift the omelet from the skillet.

5. Slide the omelet onto a large plate. Add the remaining tablespoon of butter to the skillet. Using the plate, flip the omelet over, back into the skillet, to cook the other side. Cook for another 5 minutes, or until the egg is completely set and the cheese has melted. Cut the omelet into slices and serve warm.

SWEET POTATO PEANUT STEW

coconut, sweet potatoes, garlic, chickpeas, spinach

Adding peanut butter to your stew may sound unusual at first, but trust us on this one. Peanut stew has been celebrated in western African countries for centuries, and for good reason. Made in one pot with humble ingredients, consisting of a rich, comforting broth of peanuts, sweet potatoes, tomatoes, and spices, our version of this beloved dish is like a warm hug. Feel free to swap out the fresh spinach with baby kale or up the spice factor with hot sauce of your choice. This stew can be enjoyed as is or served over brown rice for an even heartier meal.

SERVES 6 TO 8

2 tablespoons extra-virgin coconut oil

3 medium-size sweet potatoes, peeled and chopped into ½-inch cubes

½ yellow onion, diced

3 garlic cloves, minced

1 jalapeño pepper, seeded and minced

1 teaspoon curry powder

½ teaspoon ground turmeric

1 teaspoon Himalayan pink salt

1 (14-ounce) can diced tomatoes

1 (14-ounce) can coconut milk

1 (14-ounce) can chickpeas, drained and rinsed

2 cups vegetable stock

¼ cup all-natural creamy peanut butter

½ cup chopped roasted peanuts

2 cups spinach, rinsed well

TOPPINGS:

Chopped peanuts

Microgreens

Fresh cilantro

1. In a large soup pot, heat the coconut oil over medium-high heat. Add the sweet potatoes, onion, garlic, and jalapeño. Cook until a sweet potato cube is tender when poked with a fork and the onion and garlic are translucent, about 10 minutes.

2. Stir in the curry, turmeric, salt, and tomatoes and cook over medium heat for 5 minutes, or until fragrant.

3. Add the coconut milk, chickpeas, and stock and give it a good stir. Cover the pot and increase the heat to medium-high. Cook for 10 to 15 minutes, or until it comes to a low boil.

continued on page 136

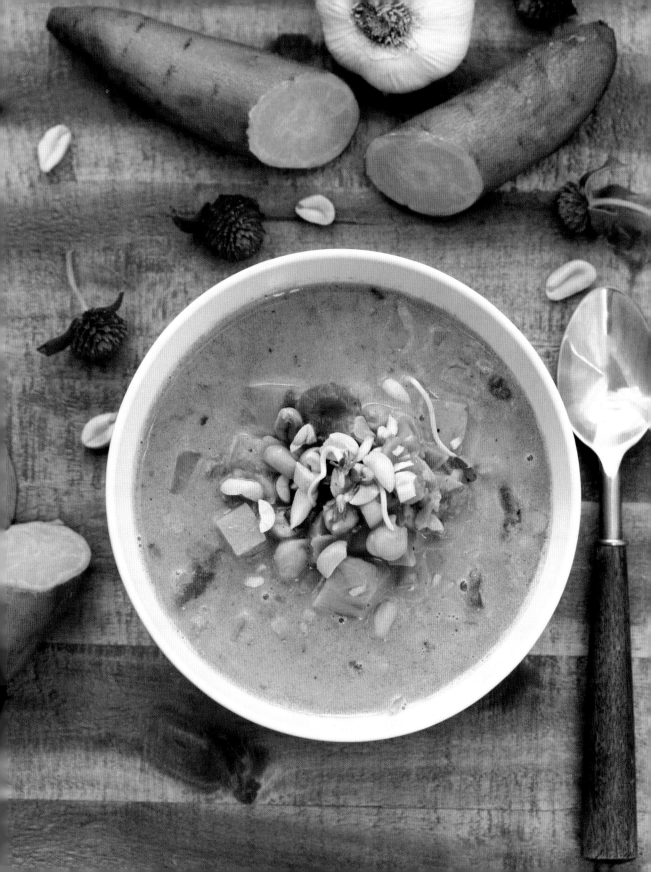

4. Stir in the peanut butter and roasted peanuts and lower the heat to medium-low. Let the stew cook for another 5 minutes.

5. Add the spinach and cook until wilted, about 1 to 2 minutes. Remove from the heat and serve immediately.

6. Top with chopped peanuts, microgreens, and cilantro. Leftovers can be stored in an airtight container for up to 3 days in the refrigerator.

PEA, PISTACHIO, AND SALMON SALAD with CARROT GINGER DRESSING

When your body is screaming for nothing but a tasty bowl of fresh greens and a light, vibrant dressing, this salad is going to hit the spot. To make this into a protein-packed meal, we top it with a beautiful fillet of salmon. Salmon is an excellent source of protein, selenium, vitamin D, and DHA for new moms. DHA is found to be essential to the development of a newborn's nervous system, and luckily DHA is easily absorbed and transferred via breast milk. The zing of ginger, the richness of salmon, the sweet crunch of sugar snap peas, and the slightly bitter notes of baby kale create a winning dinner salad that is well worth the effort. You and your baby will thank you.

CARROT GINGER DRESSING:

SERVES 6

1 teaspoon grated fresh ginger

2 carrots, peeled and chopped

1½ teaspoons red miso paste

1 shallot, chopped roughly

⅓ cup rice vinegar

½ cup sunflower oil

½ teaspoon Himalayan pink salt

SEARED SALMON:

SERVES 2

1 tablespoon extra-virgin olive oil

2 (4-ounce) fillets wild-caught salmon

Salt and freshly ground black pepper

PEA AND PISTACHIO SALAD:

SERVES 4

6 cups baby kale

⅓ cup roasted pistachios

1 cup sugar snap peas, sliced

1. Prepare the dressing: Combine all the dressing ingredients plus ⅓ cup of water in a food processor and blend for 15 seconds, or until smooth. Add more salt to taste. Set aside.

2. Prepare the salmon: Heat a skillet over medium-high heat, then heat a drizzle of olive oil in the pan.

continued on page 139

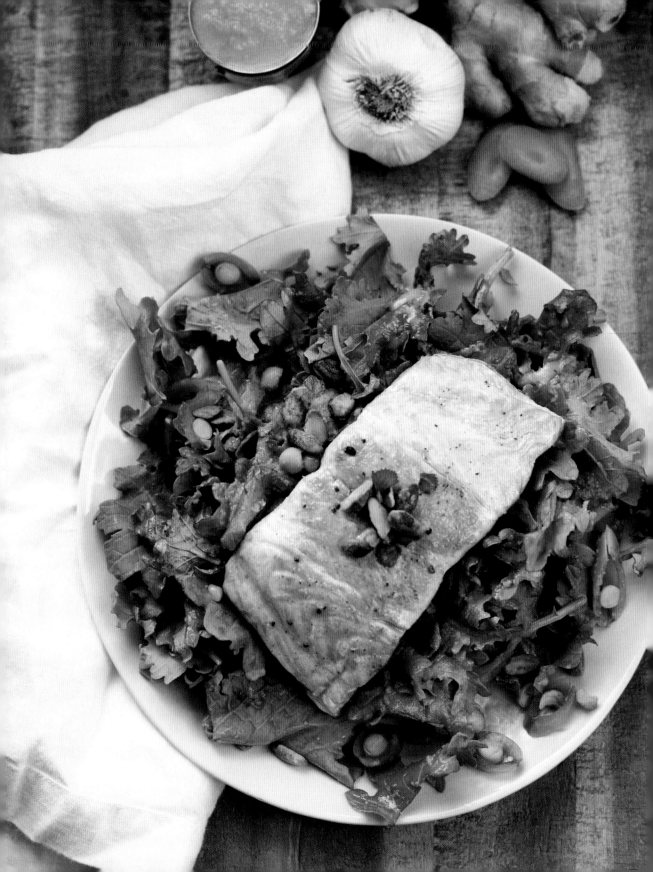

3. Season the salmon with a pinch each of salt and pepper. Place, skin side down, in the hot pan and cook it for 3 to 4 minutes, or until the color begins to lighten two thirds of the way up. Flip over to the flesh side and cook for another 2 to 3 minutes, or until evenly cooked. Remove from the heat and set aside.

4. Prepare the salad: In a large bowl, combine the baby kale, pistachios, sugar snap peas, and about ⅓ cup of the dressing and toss until well mixed. Add additional dressing, if desired. Store any remaining dressing in an airtight container in the refrigerator for up to 3 days.

5. Top the salad with the cooked salmon fillet and serve immediately.

TOM KHA CHICKPEAS

coconut milk, garlic, chickpeas, basil

Tom kha gai is one of the most beloved Thai soups, a coconut milk broth infused with aromatic herbs and fiery hot chiles. Ours uses chickpeas instead of chicken for a plant-based take on this delicious soup. For a more traditional taste, try to source the Thai ingredients from a local Asian store. If not, ginger can be substituted for the galangal, the zest of one lime in place of Kaffir lime leaves, and regular basil for Thai basil. All the aromatics do much better when they are slightly bruised to release their oils, so be sure to give the lemongrass a good whack and crack the lime leaves in half before adding them to the pot. Serve alongside steaming hot bowls of barley.

SERVES 2

4 cups canned full-fat coconut milk

1 (1-inch) knob galangal (about 1½ ounces), sliced into ¼-inch coins

2 lemongrass stalks, bruised slightly

2 garlic cloves, smashed

4 Kaffir lime leaves, cracked in half

1 to 2 Thai bird chiles (optional)

1 red bell pepper, seeded and chopped into large pieces

1 (16-ounce) can chickpeas, drained and rinsed

8 ounces fresh oyster mushrooms, stemmed

½ cup packed fresh Thai basil

Juice of 1 lime

1 to 2 teaspoons salt

1. Combine the coconut milk, galangal, lemongrass, garlic, lime leaves, and chiles, if using, in a medium-size saucepot over medium heat. Cook for 4 to 5 minutes, stirring very gently; don't let the broth come to a boil. If the broth begins to get too hot, lower the heat to low so you do not burn or curdle the coconut milk.

2. Add the bell pepper, chickpeas, and mushrooms. Cook for 3 to 4 minutes, or until the bell peppers are slightly softened.

3. Stir in the basil. Add the lime juice, 1½ teaspoons at a time, until the broth reaches your desired level of sourness. Taste and add salt until the flavors pop. Serve immediately.

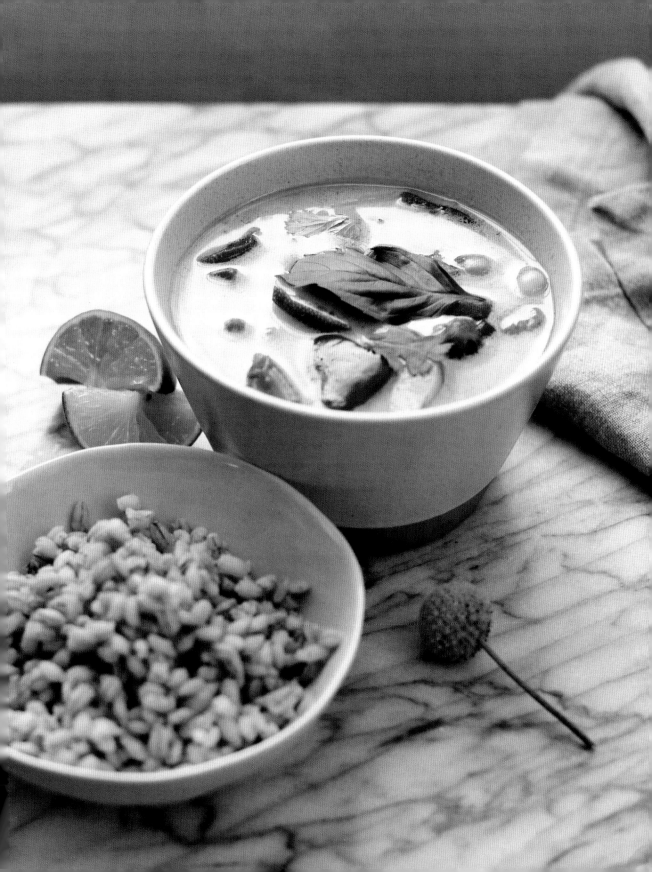

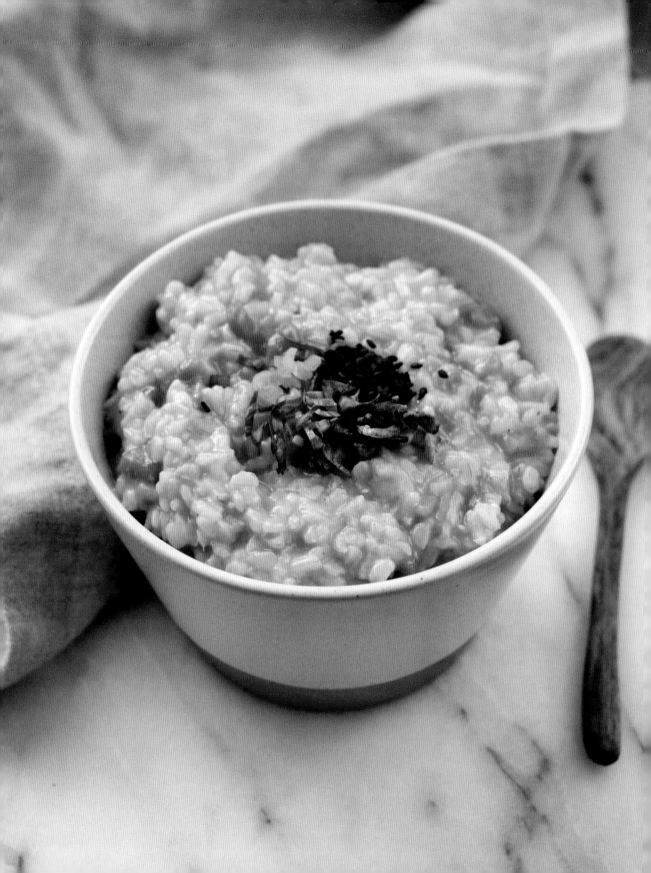

CARROT GINGER CONGEE

brown rice, carrot, nutritional yeast, ginger, black sesame seeds

Congee is a porridge made from slowly cooking rice until it breaks down and releases its starches. The result is a bowl of pure comfort. Our congee is made from brown rice and a stock that is enhanced with ginger and nutritional yeast to deliver a satisfying umami flavor. Congee is traditionally served for breakfast, but because of its long cooking time, we prefer to put it on the stove in the late afternoon and enjoy it as dinner. Of course, you can always cook it and put it in the fridge for the morning. The congee will seize up a bit as it cools. Simply loosen it up with a bit of water or stock and reheat on the stovetop.

SERVES 2 TO 4

1 cup uncooked short-grain brown rice

4 cups vegetable stock

1 large carrot, diced very small (about 1 cup)

1 tablespoon nutritional yeast

3 or 4 slices fresh ginger

OPTIONAL TOPPINGS:

Toasted black sesame seeds

Chopped scallions

Fried garlic

Soy sauce

Sesame oil

1. Rinse the brown rice in a fine-mesh sieve until the water runs clear. In a medium-size saucepan, combine the rice, stock, carrot, nutritional yeast, and ginger. Bring to a boil.

2. Cover, lower the heat to low, and let simmer for 1 hour, checking halfway through to stir and prevent any rice from sticking to the pot.

3. The congee is done when the rice and carrot are soft and the mixture has thickened to a porridge consistency. Remove the ginger slices and serve the warm congee in bowls garnished with the toppings you desire.

CRUNCHY MILLET CAKES

millet, kale, garlic, nutritional yeast

When you've got a baby, any time you can put together a quick, home-cooked meal and use one bowl and one pan, that's a huge win. If you're not familiar with millet, it is a versatile, quick-cooking grain with a slightly nutty profile. When cooked in liquid, millet softens, but when it is toasted, it becomes pleasantly crunchy. These cakes are perfect because the inside is nice and soft, but the outside develops a delicious crunch. For this reason, these are also a big hit with picky toddlers (ketchup for dipping always helps!) and a great way to sneak in some greens.

SERVES 4 TO 6

1 cup cooked millet

2 large eggs, lightly beaten

½ cup panko bread crumbs

1 cup chopped kale

2 tablespoons minced shallot

2 garlic cloves, minced

½ teaspoon salt

½ teaspoon onion powder

1 tablespoon nutritional yeast

2 tablespoons olive oil

1. Place all the ingredients, except the olive oil, in a large bowl and stir to combine. Let the batter sit for 2 to 3 minutes to allow the bread crumbs to soak up the liquid. Meanwhile, in a skillet, heat the olive oil over medium-high heat.

2. Using a ¼-cup measure, scoop up the mixture and drop it in patties into the hot oil. Lower the heat to medium.

3. Cook the millet cake for 3 to 4 minutes, or until the bottom of the cake is golden brown and crispy. With a spatula, flip the cake and cook on the other side for another 2 to 3 minutes, also until deeply golden. When the cake is golden and crisped on both sides, transfer it to a paper towel–lined plate to soak up any excess oil. Repeat with the remaining batter until all the millet cakes are prepared. Serve immediately.

Serving suggestions: Top with a dollop of Greek yogurt and lemon zest. We also like to serve these on a bed of arugula simply dressed with lemon, olive oil, salt, and pepper.

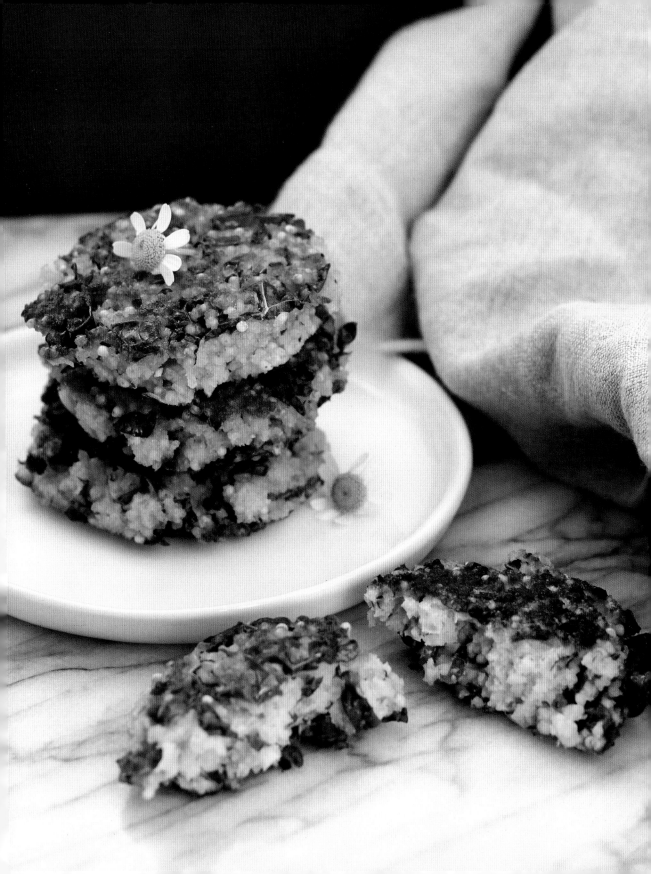

Treats

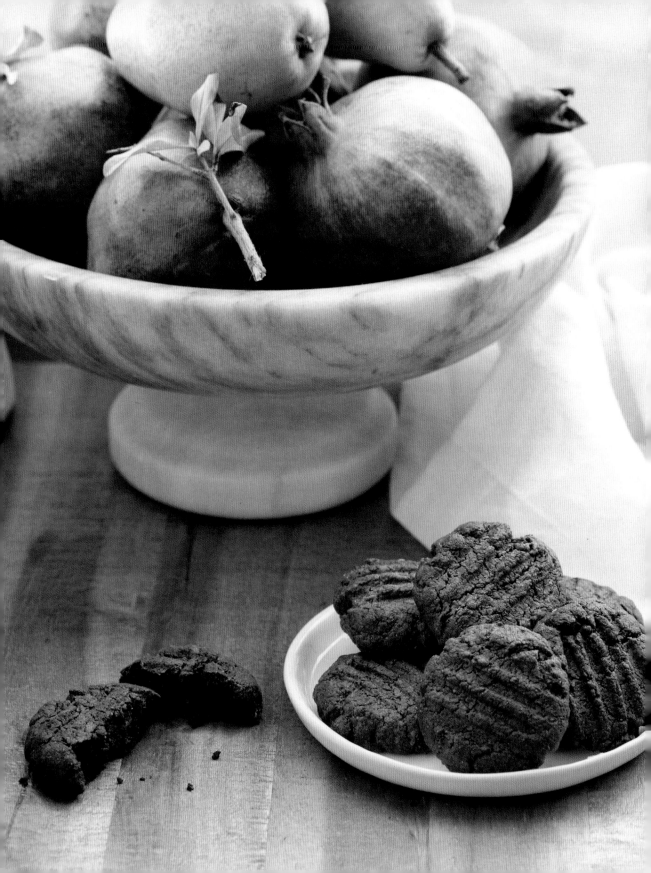

FLOURLESS CHOCOLATE ALMOND BUTTER COOKIES

almonds

You may have tried a flourless chocolate cake before; well, here's a flourless chocolate cookie for you. Not only is this cookie naturally gluten-free, but it has no refined oils or butter, only natural healthy fats from the almond butter. Almonds are an ideal food for breastfeeding because they are so high in healthy fats. In fact, some studies show they keep you feeling full longer due to their high protein and fiber content. Yes, these are still cookies, but the magnesium in almonds helps manage blood sugar levels, so you're less likely to feel that sugar crash.

MAKES ABOUT 18 COOKIES

1 large egg

1 cup coconut sugar

1 cup crunchy unsalted almond butter

¼ cup unsweetened cocoa powder

1 teaspoon baking soda

¼ teaspoon fine-grain sea salt

½ teaspoon almond extract

½ teaspoon pure vanilla extract

¼ cup mini dark chocolate chips

1. Preheat the oven to 350°F. Line a rimmed cookie sheet with parchment paper.

2. In a medium-size bowl, lightly beat the egg and coconut sugar together until combined.

3. Mix in the almond butter until incorporated, then stir in the cocoa, baking soda, salt, and almond and vanilla extracts. Mix until incorporated. Stir in mini dark chocolate chips.

4. Scoop the dough by tablespoons and roll into 1-inch balls. Place the balls 1 inch apart on the prepared cookie sheet. Use a fork or the palm of your hand to gently flatten the dough into disks.

5. Bake for 11 to 13 minutes, or until the cookies are set and the tops are slightly cracked. Remove from the oven and transfer to a wire rack to cool. Leftover cookies can be stored in an airtight container for up to 3 days.

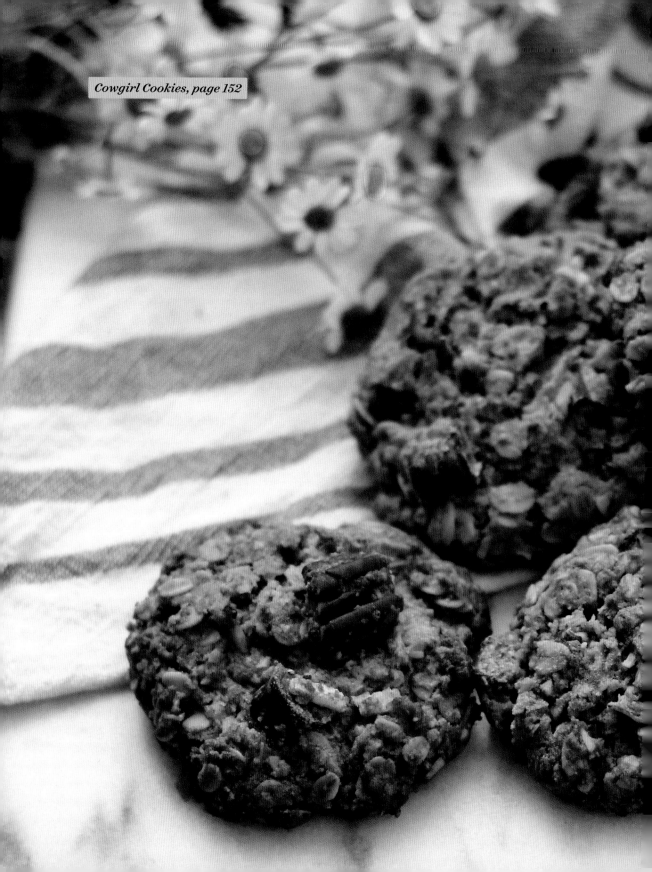
Cowgirl Cookies, page 152

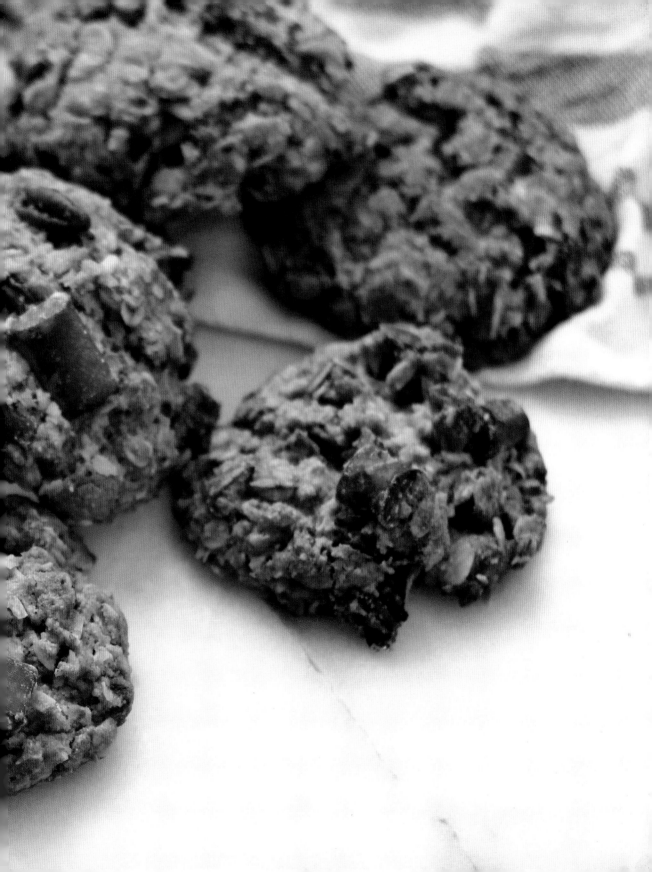

COWGIRL COOKIES

almonds, oats, brewer's yeast

A cowboy cookie is a chocolate chip cookie that is made chewier by adding oats, pecans, and coconut. Our cowgirl version is decidedly more mama-friendly with the addition of brewer's yeast, dark chocolate chunks, and a sprinkling of pink salt.

MAKES 2 DOZEN COOKIES

½ cup almond flour

¾ cup organic oat flour

¼ cup debittered brewer's yeast

½ teaspoon baking soda

½ teaspoon Himalayan pink salt or sea salt

10 tablespoons (1¼ sticks, 5 ounces) unsalted grass-fed butter

1¼ cups dark brown sugar

1 large egg

2 teaspoons pure vanilla extract

2 cups organic old-fashioned rolled oats

1 cup pecans, roughly chopped

1 cup shredded unsweetened coconut

¾ cup dark chocolate chips

1. Preheat the oven to 350°F and line a rimmed baking sheet with parchment paper.

2. In a medium-size bowl, mix together the flours, brewer's yeast, baking soda, and salt. Set aside.

3. In the bowl of a stand mixer fitted with the paddle attachment, beat the butter and brown sugar together until smooth, about 3 minutes. Add the egg and vanilla and beat until incorporated.

4. On a slow setting, carefully pour the flour mixture into the butter mixture. Add the oats, pecans, coconut, and chocolate chips and mix until just incorporated, but be careful not to overmix the dough.

5. Scoop the dough by rounded tablespoons and form into balls (each should be about 2 tablespoons of dough). Place the balls 2 inches apart on the prepared cookie sheet. Gently press down the balls with your hands, or the back of a table-spoon, to lightly flatten.

6. Bake for 12 to 14 minutes, or until the edges are deeply golden. Remove from the oven and transfer to a wire rack to cool. Leftover cookies can be stored in an airtight container for up to 3 days.

COOKIE DOUGH BITES

almonds, brewer's yeast, coconut oil

Who says you can't have your lactation cookie dough and eat it, too? These are simple and deceptively delicious little bites to stock your fridge with right before Baby arrives. We say "deceptive" because they taste so indulgent yet they're packed with all good things. You may want to double the recipe . . .

MAKES ABOUT 16 BITES

1 cup unsweetened shredded coconut

½ cup almond flour

1 teaspoon debittered brewer's yeast

1 tablespoon extra-virgin coconut oil

1 tablespoon pure maple syrup

1 teaspoon pure vanilla extract

¼ teaspoon Himalayan pink salt or sea salt

1 tablespoon mini chocolate chips

1. Place all the ingredients into a food processor and pulse about ten times, or until the mixture begins to come together into a ball.

2. Scoop by heaping tablespoons and roll into 1-inch balls with your hands.

3. Place the cookie dough bites in the refrigerator to chill for at least 10 minutes to firm up before enjoying. Keep the bites refrigerated in an airtight container.

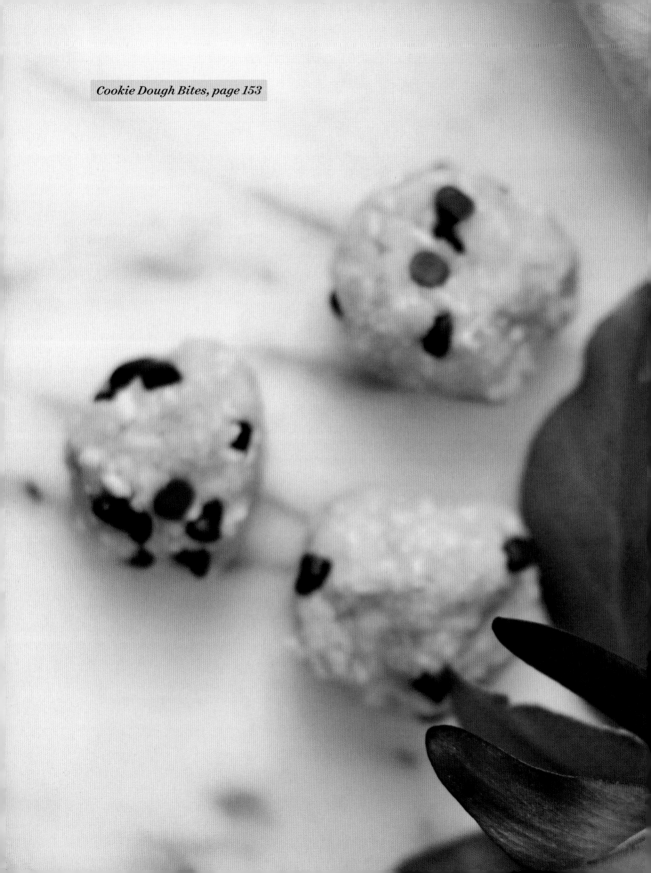

Cookie Dough Bites, page 153

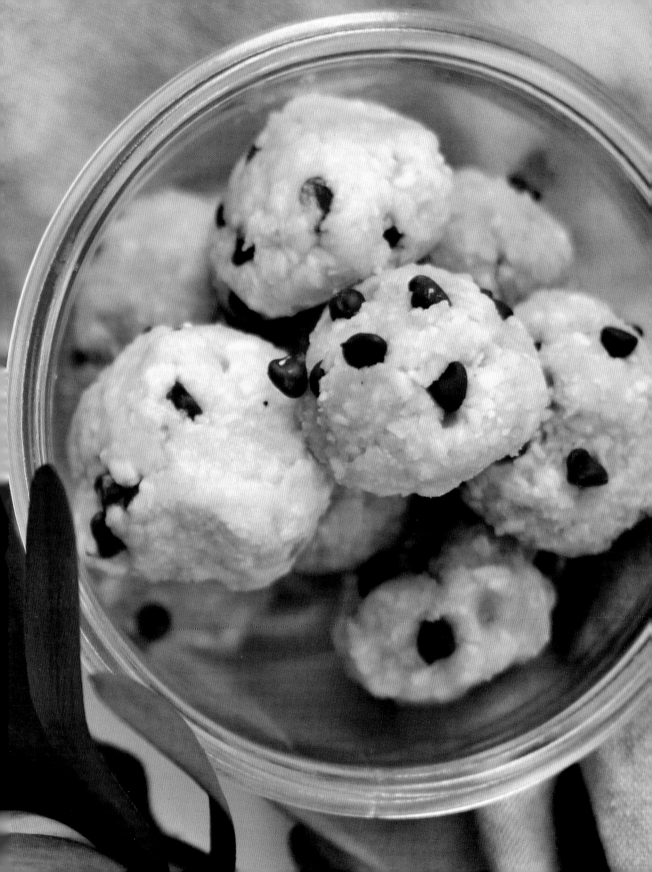

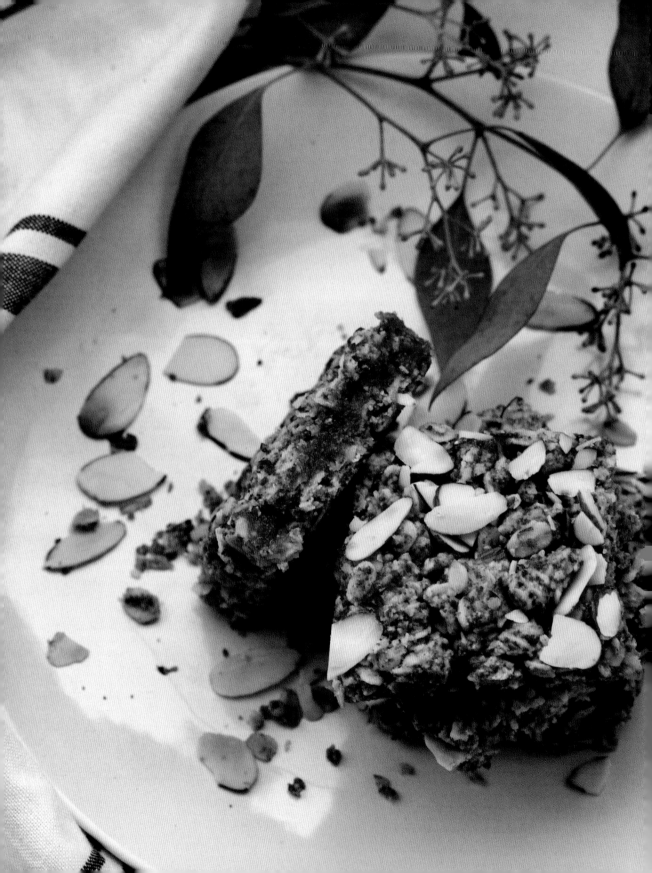

APRICOT OAT SQUARES

oats, coconut, apricot, chia seeds, almonds

Here's a take on an old family recipe in our house, date bars. They had a crumble topping made from butter, brown sugar, oats, and white flour, and the middle was filled with gooey cooked dates. None of the kids ever complained about the flavor, but when we tried eating them as adults, wow, are they sweet! In our version, we swapped white flour for whole wheat, cut the sugar in half, and swapped the sticky sweet dates for a tart apricot jam. We also upped the protein with chia seeds and almonds. This version seems to be just right for us adults and kids are still not complaining.

MAKES 9 SQUARES

Extra-virgin coconut oil, for pan

1 cup organic old-fashioned rolled oats

1 cup whole wheat pastry flour

⅓ cup coconut sugar

¼ cup unsweetened shredded coconut

¼ teaspoon baking soda

⅛ teaspoon salt

½ cup extra-virgin coconut oil, melted

½ cup plus 2 tablespoons apricot jam

1 teaspoon chia seeds

⅓ cup sliced almonds

1. Preheat the oven to 350°F and grease an 8-inch square baking pan with the coconut oil.

2. In a medium-size bowl, combine the oats, flour, coconut sugar, shredded coconut, baking soda, and salt.

3. Add the melted coconut oil and mix until the mixture comes together into coarse crumbs.

4. Pour half of the crumb mixture (about 1½ cups) into the prepared baking pan. Spread the crumbs evenly on the bottom of the pan. Press down gently with your fingers to form an even bottom crust.

5. Add the apricot jam. Carefully spread the jam over the crust, using the back of a spoon or a butter knife. To prevent the jam from burning on the edges, leave a

continued on page 158

¼-inch border jam-free all around. Sprinkle the chia seeds on the jam and then top with the remaining crumble mixture and sliced almonds.

6. Give the pan a good jiggle back and forth to let everything settle, and press down the top lightly so the toppings stick to the jam.

7. Bake for 35 to 40 minutes, or until the oats and almonds are toasty brown and fragrant. Remove from the oven and let the bars cool in the baking pan before slicing and serving. Store any leftovers in an airtight container at room temperature for up to 2 days.

DARK CHOCOLATE BUCKWHEAT BANANA BREAD

buckwheat, Greek yogurt

This quick bread is a wonderful treat to slice into on a rainy, foggy day and enjoy alongside a steaming mug of Earl Grey tea. Imagine Baby is sweetly napping while you regain your breath and sanity with a quiet moment to yourself. At least that's how we picture it in our minds . . . No matter how you serve it, there is something very cozy and comforting about this classic quick bread that feels like an old friend. Just a few moments of mommy-time can help relax and recharge you for another day of nurturing.

MAKES 1 LOAF

8 tablespoons (1 stick, 4 ounces) unsalted grass-fed butter

1 cup coconut sugar

2 large eggs

1 teaspoon pure vanilla extract

1 cup whole wheat pastry flour

½ cup buckwheat flour

1 teaspoon baking soda

½ teaspoon salt

3 overripe bananas, mashed

½ cup full-fat Greek yogurt

½ cup dark chocolate chips

1. Preheat the oven to 350°F. Grease a 9 by 5-inch loaf pan.

2. In a small saucepan on the stovetop over low heat or in a microwave-safe dish in the microwave, warm the butter until just melted.

3. In a bowl, combine the coconut sugar and melted butter. Whisk in the eggs and vanilla.

4. In a separate bowl, combine the flours, baking soda, and salt.

5. Mix the dry ingredients into the wet until just combined.

6. Fold in the mashed bananas, yogurt, and chocolate chips.

7. Pour into the prepared loaf pan and bake for 50 to 55 minutes, or until a toothpick inserted into the middle of the loaf comes out clean. Remove from the oven and transfer to a wire rack to cool. Leftovers can be stored in an airtight container for up to 3 days.

Dark Chocolate Buckwheat Banana Bread, page 159

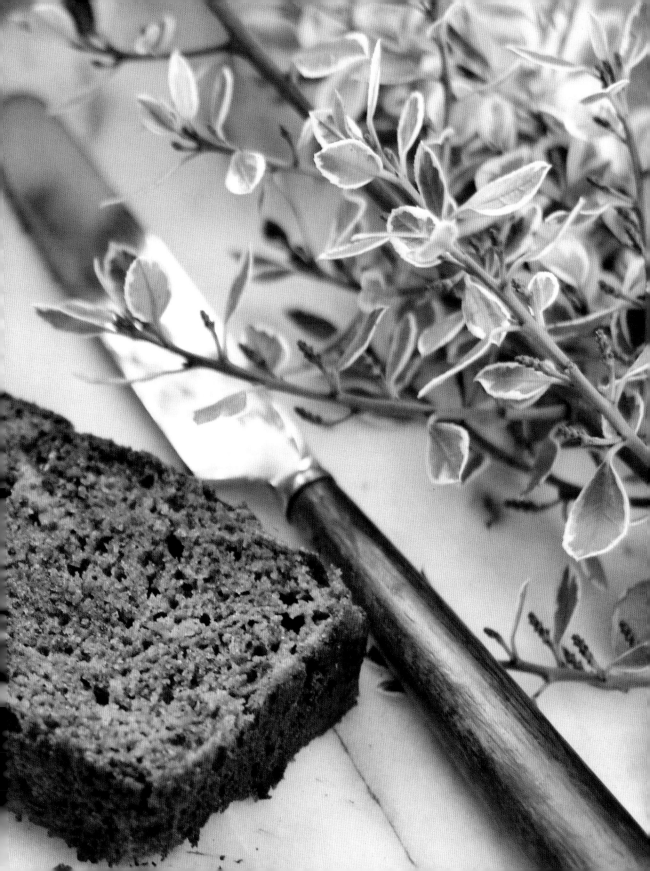

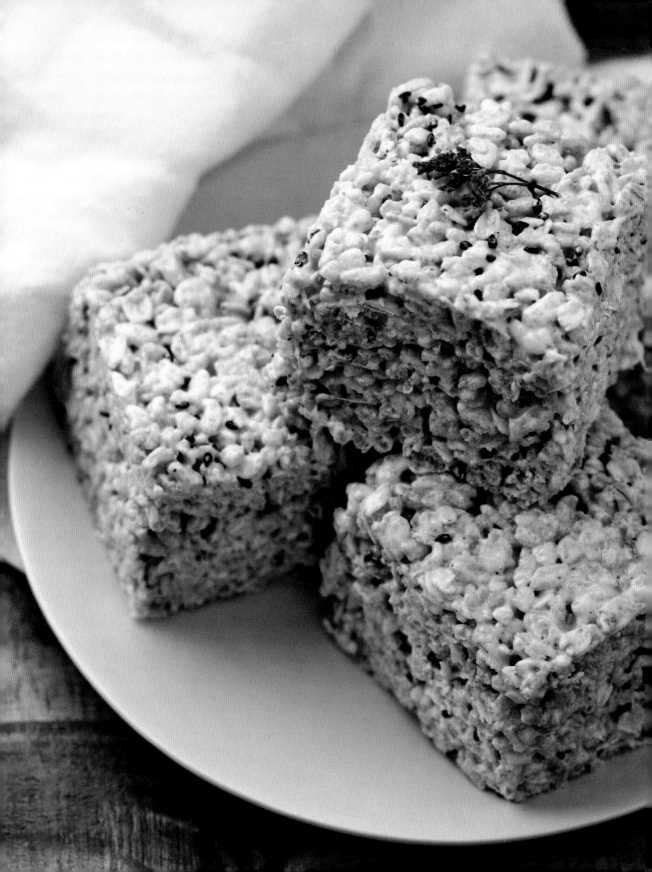

OATMEAL CRISPY TREATS

oats, brown rice, brewer's yeast, coconut oil, black sesame seeds

Our grandma always added oats to our crispy treats growing up, and we never thought twice about it. It wasn't until adulthood that we realized that was her own special "touch." Now when thinking of treats with oats, of course, grandma's recipe comes to mind. The oats add a chewy texture to complement the crunch of the crispy rice and lend a more whole-grain flavor overall. We've also added brewer's yeast and sesame seeds to increase the lactation quotient. The end result is, dare we say, better than the originals.

MAKES ABOUT 9 SERVINGS

1 cup organic old-fashioned rolled oats

5 cups brown crispy rice cereal

1 tablespoon debittered brewer's yeast

3 tablespoons extra-virgin coconut oil

5 cups all-natural mini marshmallows

1 tablespoon black sesame seeds

¾ teaspoon Himalayan pink salt

1. Grease a 9-inch square baking pan and set aside.

2. In a large bowl, combine the oats, rice cereal, and brewer's yeast and mix well.

3. In a large pot over medium-low heat, melt together the coconut oil and marshmallows, stirring frequently so the mixture doesn't brown on the bottom.

4. Once the marshmallows are just melted, remove from the heat. Pour the cereal mixture into the melted marshmallow mixture, along with the black sesame seeds and salt. Stir until fully incorporated.

5. Pour the mixture into the prepared baking pan, pressing down gently with a large greased spoon, or a spatula, to flatten.

6. Allow to set for 10 minutes. Cut into nine squares and store in an airtight container for up to a week.

LACTATION ENERGY BITES

oatmeal, coconut, brewer's yeast

The only problem with lactation cookies is that you have to wait for them to bake and then wait for them to cool. Not feeling up to waiting? Go the Lactation Energy Bite route. They deliver that sweet taste and chew of a cookie but come together in minutes in a food processor. Energy bites are also gluten-free (if using certified GF oats) and egg-free, and don't contain any refined sugars, so they work with a lot of different lifestyles. These are highly customizable with different nut butters and dried fruits, but this is the recipe we always end up coming back to in our house.

MAKES ABOUT 20 BITES

8 pitted dates

3 tablespoons all-natural unsalted creamy peanut butter

¼ cup organic old-fashioned rolled oats

3 tablespoons unsweetened shredded coconut

1 tablespoon debittered brewer's yeast

¼ teaspoon pure vanilla extract

Pinch of Himalayan pink salt

1. Place all the ingredients in a food processor and process for 30 seconds, scraping down the sides of the blender with a spatula as needed, until a chunky dough forms.

2. Scoop the dough by rounded ½ tablespoons and roll into ½-inch balls with your hands.

3. Store in an airtight container in the refrigerator for up to a week.

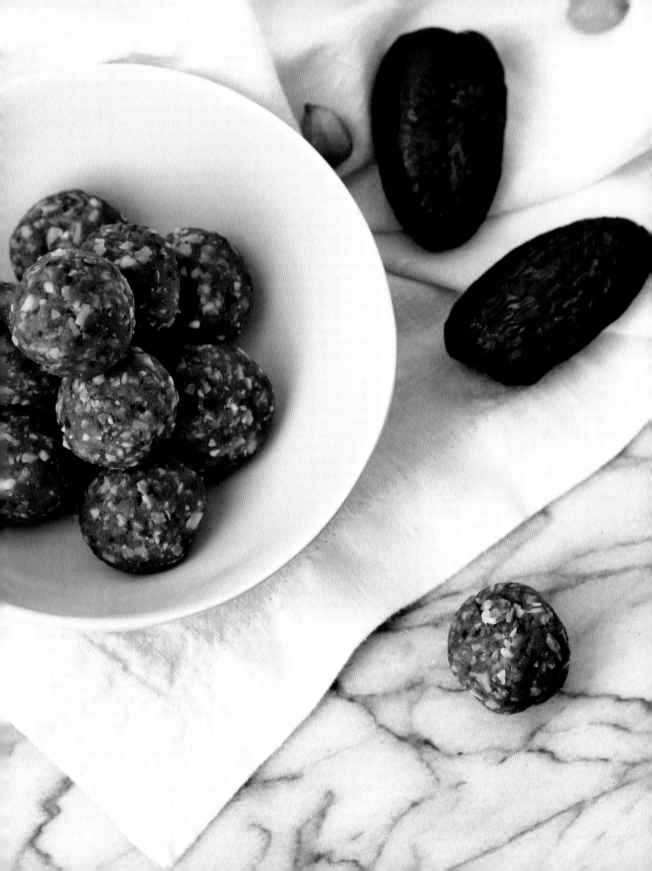

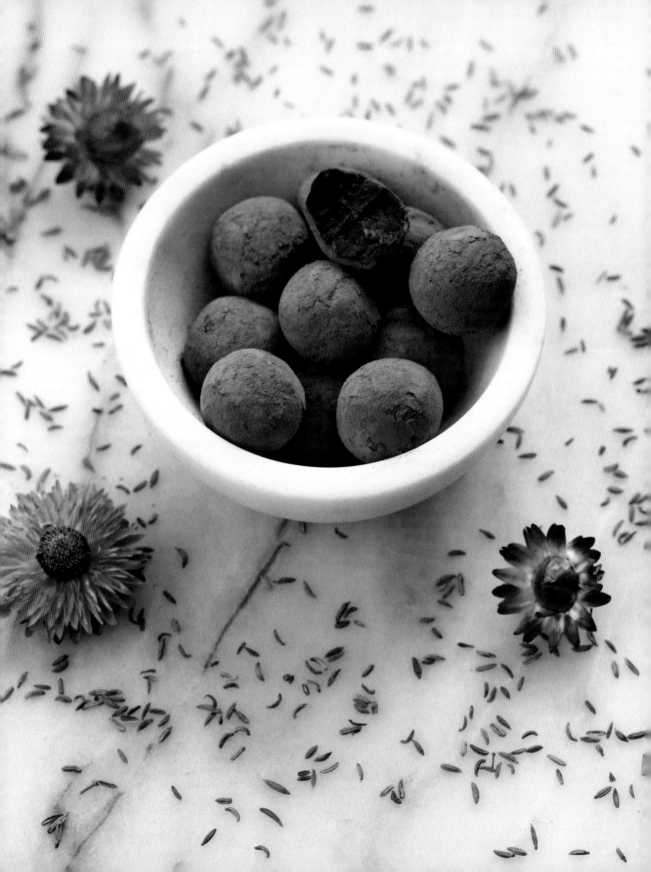

COCOA ANISE TRUFFLES

aniseeds

We guess either you're an anise lover or you're not, and honestly we never put ourselves in the black licorice camp. Yet, when we had these, they really blew our minds, and we've become a little bit obsessed—so even if you're not a licorice fan, we say give these indulgent truffles a chance. They are a cinch to throw together, and their smooth, rich decadence will satisfy your every sweet tooth and chocolate craving. Sugar and dairy need not apply. Who knew?

MAKES ABOUT 12 TRUFFLES

½ cup packed, pitted dates (about 6 dates)

4 teaspoons unsweetened cocoa powder, plus 3 tablespoons for rolling

½ teaspoon extra-virgin coconut oil

¼ teaspoon pure vanilla extract

¼ teaspoon aniseeds

Pinch of salt

1. Place all the ingredients, except the extra cocoa powder, in a food processor. Pulse the mixture until smooth, scraping down the sides as needed.

2. Scoop the truffle mixture by ½ tablespoons and roll into ½-inch balls. If the mixture is sticky, lightly dampen your hands with water before rolling.

3. Roll the balls in the reserved cocoa powder to coat. Enjoy cold or at room temperature. Store in an airtight container in the fridge for up to 3 days.

DARK CHOCOLATE FIG ALMOND BARK

figs, almonds, buckwheat, hemp seeds

Chocolate bark is basically a chocolate bar, but thinner and smaller and with a bunch of yummy, healthy add-ins. It's incredibly easy to make and very impressive-looking. It makes a really beautiful and thoughtful gift to share at baby showers and deliver to new and expecting mamas. Our bark is a glorious combination of dried fruits and nuts with crunchy bits from the buckwheat groats. A few pieces of this bark is all you'll need to satisfy an after-dinner sweet craving.

MAKES 12 TO 14 SERVINGS

1 cup dark chocolate chips

2 dried figs, chopped small

¼ cup chopped roasted almonds

2 teaspoons uncooked buckwheat groats

1 teaspoon hemp seeds

1 tablespoon bee pollen (optional)

1. Line a rimmed baking sheet with waxed paper or parchment paper and set aside.

2. Melt the dark chocolate chips in a microwave-safe bowl in the microwave in 20-second intervals until melted and smooth, but be careful not to overheat or the chocolate may burn or seize.

3. Stir in the chopped figs and almonds. Give it a good stir until the figs and almonds are well coated.

4. Pour the chocolate onto the prepared baking sheet and spread to about a ¼-inch thickness. Sprinkle with the buckwheat groats, hemp seeds, and bee pollen, if using.

5. Store in an airtight container for up to 2 weeks.

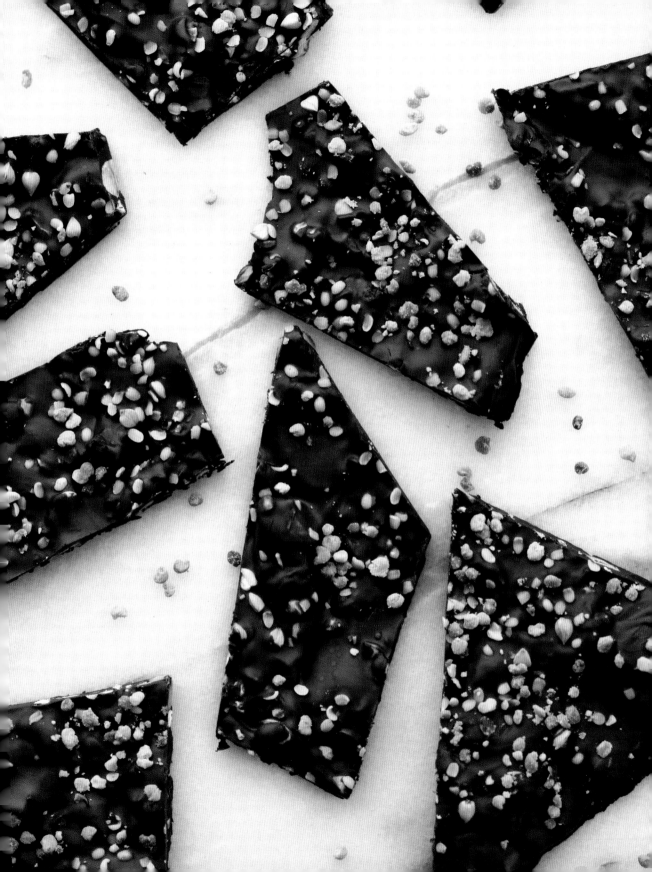

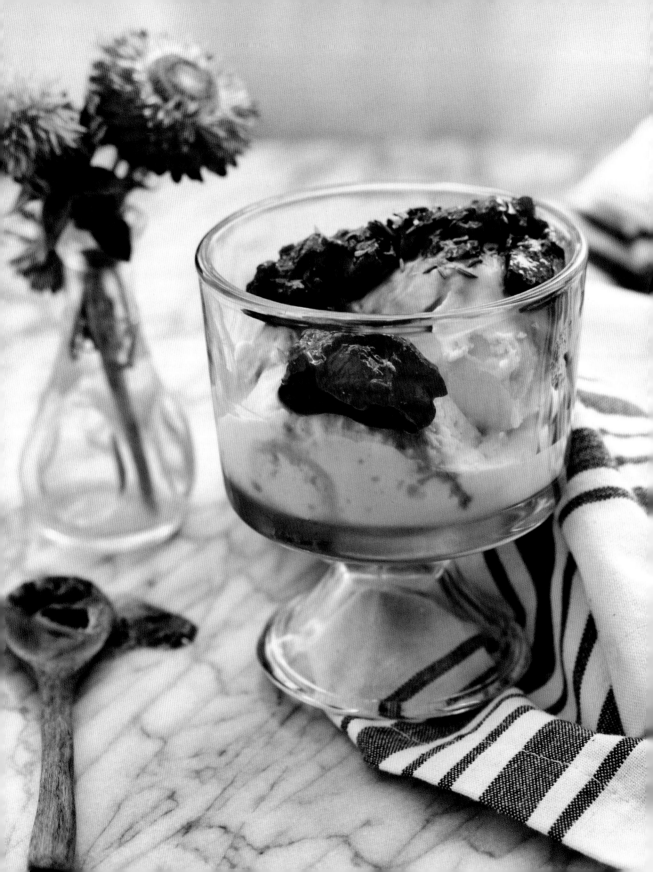

SIMPLE STEWED APRICOTS

Plump and juicy with a complex sweetness from the coconut sugar and anise syrup, these stewed apricots are a delight. You can enjoy them warm, spooned over vanilla ice cream or cake, or cold straight from the fridge. They make a wonderful addition to yogurt or muesli, and a spoonful will take a plain bowl of warm steel-cut oats to new heights.

MAKES 2 CUPS STEWED APRICOTS

1 cup dried unsulfured apricots

⅓ cup coconut sugar

1 tablespoon aniseeds

1. Combine all the ingredients plus 3 cups of water in a medium-size saucepan and place over high heat.

2. Bring to a boil, then lower the heat to low and cover. Simmer for 20 to 25 minutes, or until the apricots are plump and the remaining liquid has thickened to a syrup.

3. Remove from the heat and let cool for 5 minutes.

4. Serve warm, or allow the apricots to cool completely and store in an airtight container in the fridge for up to 1 week.

COCONUT CARAMEL DIPPERS

coconut milk, nutritional yeast

Making your own caramel is a lot easier than you might imagine. Just pop some milk and sugar in a pot and simmer until it turns into creamy caramel. Voilà! Coconut sugar caramel has a richer, deeper, more complex flavor than traditional milk caramels made from white sugar. Because nutritional yeast lends a nutty, buttery richness to sweets, it puts this already mouthwatering caramel sauce over the top. We like to dip some tart, crisp apple slices in and cover them with chopped peanuts.

SERVES 4

1 (14-ounce) can full-fat coconut milk

½ cup coconut sugar

1 teaspoon nutritional yeast

⅛ teaspoon pure vanilla extract

TO SERVE:

3 or 4 large apples, cored and sliced

¼ cup crushed peanuts

1. In a small saucepan, combine the coconut milk and coconut sugar and bring to a boil over medium-high heat.

2. Lower the heat to low and simmer at a soft boil for 30 to 35 minutes, stirring occasionally to break up any bits.

3. When the mixture is thickened and glossy and can coat the back of a spoon, remove from the heat. Whisk in the nutritional yeast and vanilla and continue to whisk until the yeast flakes have dissolved.

4. Serve warm, or let cool. The caramel sauce will thicken more as it cools. Serve with apple slices and crushed peanuts for dipping. Store the caramel in an airtight container in the refrigerator for up to 2 weeks.

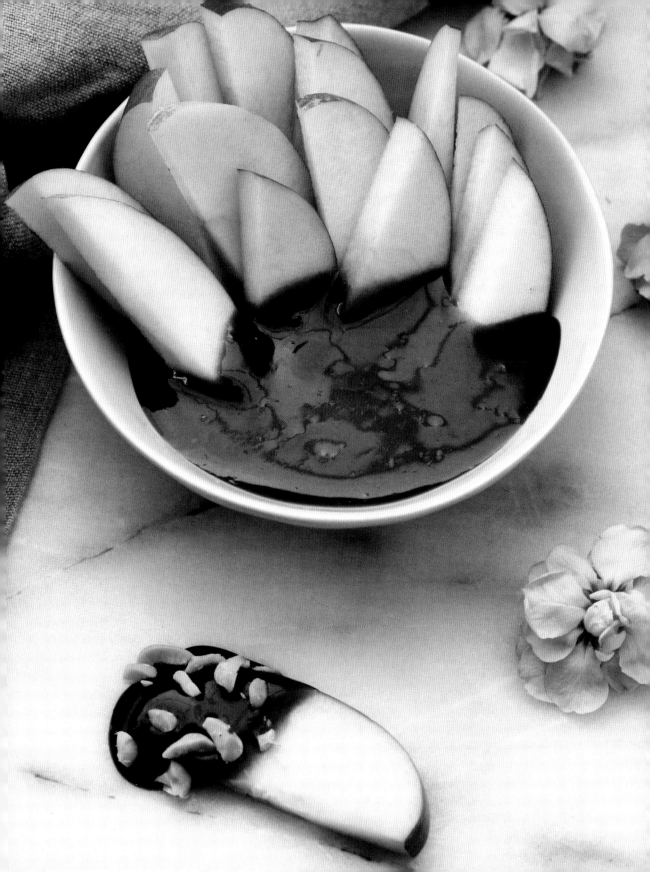

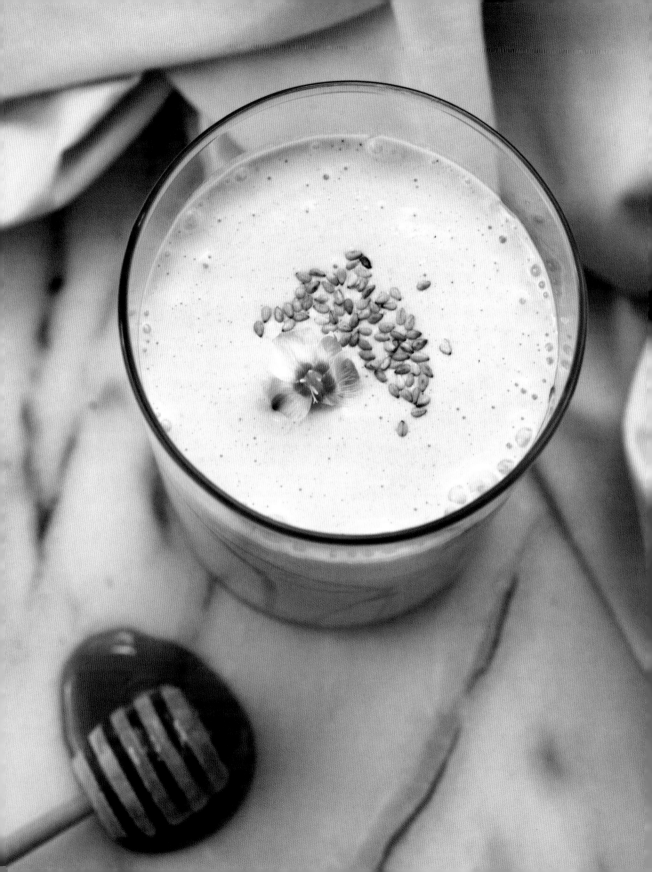

SALTED TAHINI MILK SHAKES

almond milk, tahini, brewer's yeast

After visiting our local ice-cream parlor and trying—and loving—its honeycomb flavor, it got us thinking. If honey and ice cream are an amazing combo, and sesame and honey are, too, then what are we waiting for? Let's get this tahini and honey milk shake party started. And boy, it does not disappoint. The brewer's yeast and salt provide the right balance of savory with the sweet notes of honey and nuttiness of tahini. It leaves you wanting more; we'll just leave it at that.

SERVES 2

1 cup vanilla gelato or ice cream (dairy or dairy-free both work well)

⅓ cup unsweetened vanilla almond milk

¼ cup tahini

3 teaspoons honey

1½ teaspoons debittered brewer's yeast

Scant ¼ teaspoon kosher salt

Place all the ingredients in a blender and blend until smooth, about 15 seconds. Pour into two tall glasses and serve immediately.

LACTATION ICE POPS

fennel seeds, raspberry leaves, nettle leaves

Here's to all those summer babies and moms giving birth at the height of the heat. There is something nostalgic about ice pops that reminds us of being nursed back to health as kids ourselves. (Our moms gave us frozen pops when we had a sore throat or when we were in the hospital getting our tonsils out.) These lactation tea pops make for a comforting treat to have on hand in the freezer for after birth. We tossed a few fresh raspberries into ours, but blueberries or strawberry slices would also be lovely.

MAKES 4 POPS

1 cup DIY Lactation Iced Tea
(page 193)

2 tablespoons orange juice, or
favorite juice of your choice

1 to 2 tablespoons agave syrup or
monkfruit sweetener, or to taste

6 to 8 raspberries

1. In a liquid measuring cup, stir together the lactation tea and juice. Stir in your preferred sweetener to taste.

2. Pour into four ice pop molds and add one or two berries to each mold. Freeze for 3 hours, or until frozen.

3. Carefully remove the pops from the molds and store in an airtight container in the freezer for up to a month.

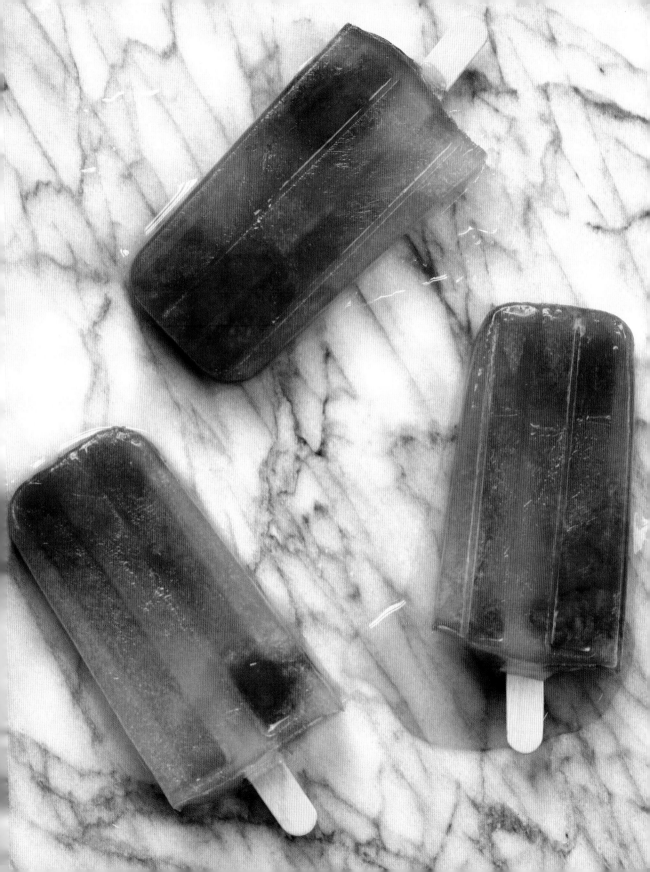

Drinks

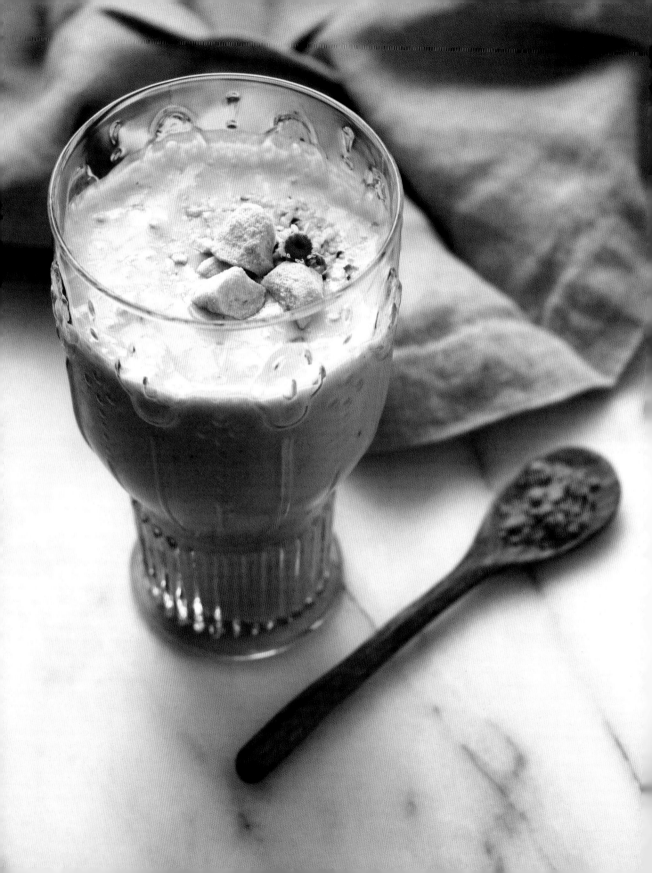

GOLDEN MILK SMOOTHIE

coconut, ginger, hemp seeds

A root related to ginger, turmeric has not been widely used in the Western diet. A quick Internet search will yield hundreds of articles about the health benefits of turmeric and its antioxidant, anti-inflammatory substance, curcumin. With significant research highlighting its positive effects on everything from cancer prevention to memory, we are all in agreement that turmeric is an excellent addition to a healthy postpartum diet. If you are turmeric-shy, or are just not sure how to incorporate it, start with this creamy, not-too-sweet smoothie and you'll be a convert.

SERVES 1

1 cup coconut milk or almond milk

1 ripe banana, frozen

1 teaspoon ground turmeric

½ teaspoon grated fresh ginger

1 tablespoon hemp seeds

Pinch of ground black pepper

1 teaspoon MCT oil or extra-virgin coconut oil

Place all the ingredients in a blender and blend until smooth. Pour into a glass and serve.

Serving suggestions: Top with additional hemp seeds, freeze-dried mango, or coconut flakes.

WARM SPICED MOLASSES

cashew milk, ginger, molasses

Warm, sweet, and creamy, this comforting drink can be enjoyed during your evening pump, or with your breakfast in place of coffee. It has a sweet, earthy richness from the blackstrap molasses. Unlike other sugars, molasses is rich in calcium and iron. Cinnamon and ginger both have anti-inflammatory properties, making this a welcome addition to your postpartum routine. On a hot day, you can omit the cinnamon and ginger and store in the fridge to enjoy later over ice as a sweet afternoon treat.

SERVES 1

1 cup cashew milk, or milk of your
  choice

1 cinnamon stick

1 (1-inch) piece fresh ginger, cut into
  4 or 5 thin slices

1½ teaspoons to 1 tablespoon
  unsulfured blackstrap molasses

1. In a small saucepan over medium heat, combine the milk, cinnamon stick, and ginger slices. Bring to a gentle boil, then lower the heat to low and let simmer for 5 minutes.

2. Remove from the heat and stir in 1½ teaspoons of the molasses. Give it a taste. If you prefer a stronger molasses flavor, continue adding a little bit at a time until you reach your desired sweetness. Remove the cinnamon stick and ginger slices before serving and enjoy warm.

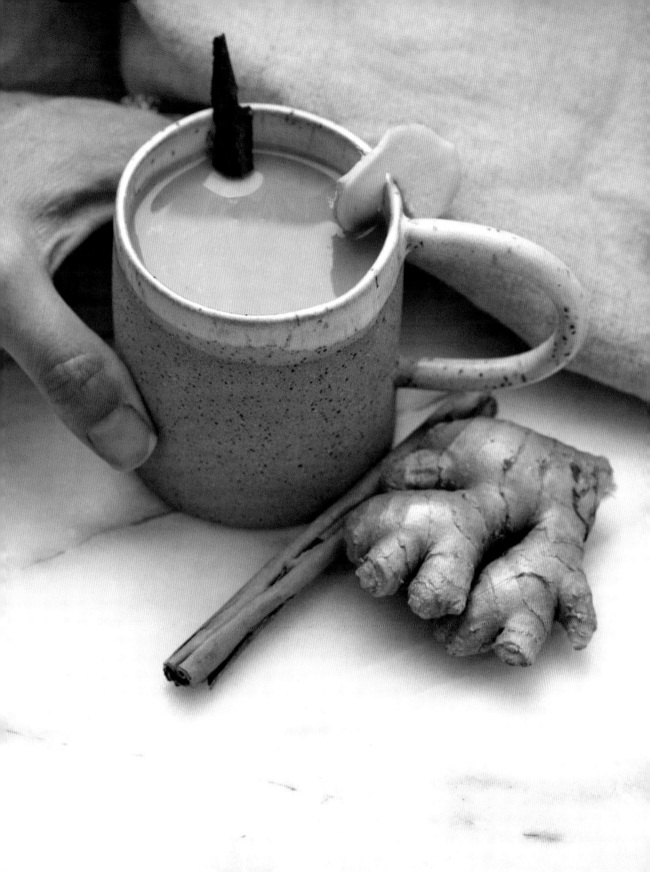

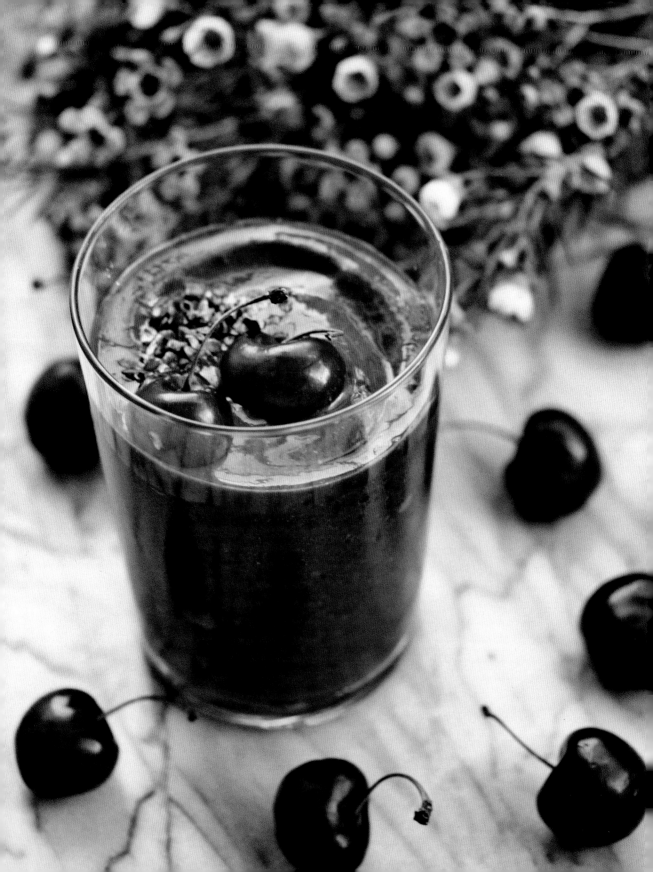

CHOCOLATE CHERRY SMOOTHIE

almond, coconut, flaxseeds, brewer's yeast

Brewer's yeast can be a tricky ingredient to work with because of its savory, bitter profile. That's why lots of lactation smoothies out there are flat-out hard to drink. Breastfeeding is difficult enough without having to choke down unpleasant smoothies! However, when paired with other strong flavors, such as sweet cherries and earthy cocoa powder, brewer's yeast shines. It helps bring out a savory note to balance all the others and make a not-too-sweet, grown-up smoothie you'll actually look forward to drinking. Promise.

SERVES 1

2 cups frozen dark cherries

⅓ cup almond milk

⅓ cup coconut milk

1 tablespoon unsweetened cocoa powder

1 tablespoon flaxseeds

1 teaspoon debittered brewer's yeast

Place all the ingredients into a blender and blend until smooth. Pour into a glass and enjoy immediately.

Serving suggestion: Top with cacao nibs and fresh or frozen cherries.

TURMERIC CARROT TONIC

carrots, turmeric

You don't need a juicer to enjoy fresh, made-to-order juices at home. All you need is a blender and some cheesecloth. A high-powered blender is best, but a conventional one will get the job done. So, what are you waiting for? Even though this may be your fourth day of not leaving the house, this invigorating turmeric carrot tonic will make you feel like you're at a trendy LA juice shop. Not to mention, making your own juice at home is an enormous savings. More money to put toward cute baby clothes!

SERVES 1

3 organic carrots, peeled and cut into 1-inch chunks

1 (2-inch) knob fresh turmeric, peeled and cut into 1-inch chunks

1 cup freshly squeezed tangerine juice

1. Combine the carrot and turmeric chunks and the juice in a blender and blend until liquefied.

2. Place a piece of cheesecloth over the mouth of a bowl. Gently pour the carrot mixture onto the cheesecloth. Lift and gather up all sides of the cheesecloth and squeeze the juice through, keeping the pulp inside the cheesecloth. Repeat until all the juice is strained through the cheesecloth. Discard the pulp. Enjoy immediately.

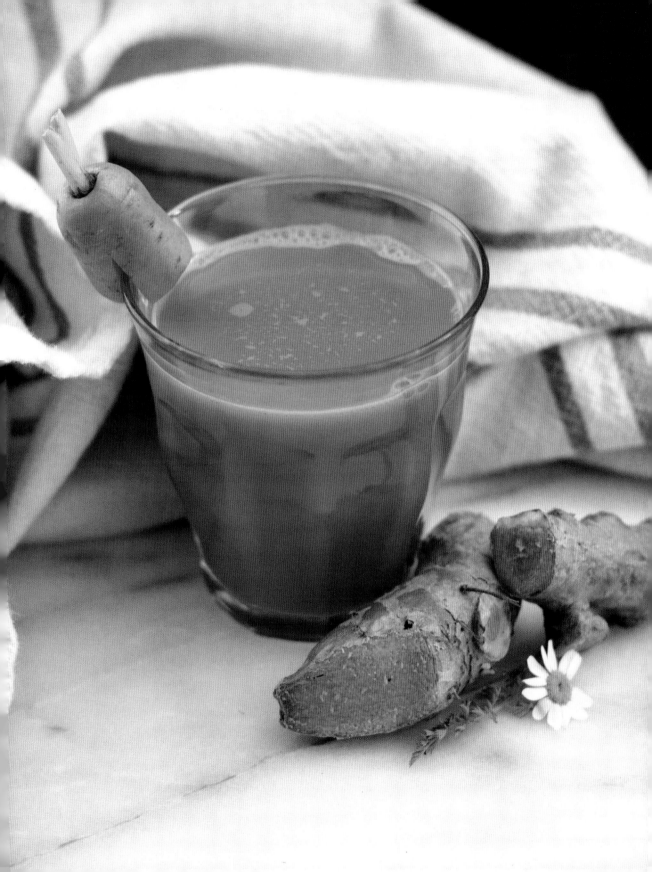

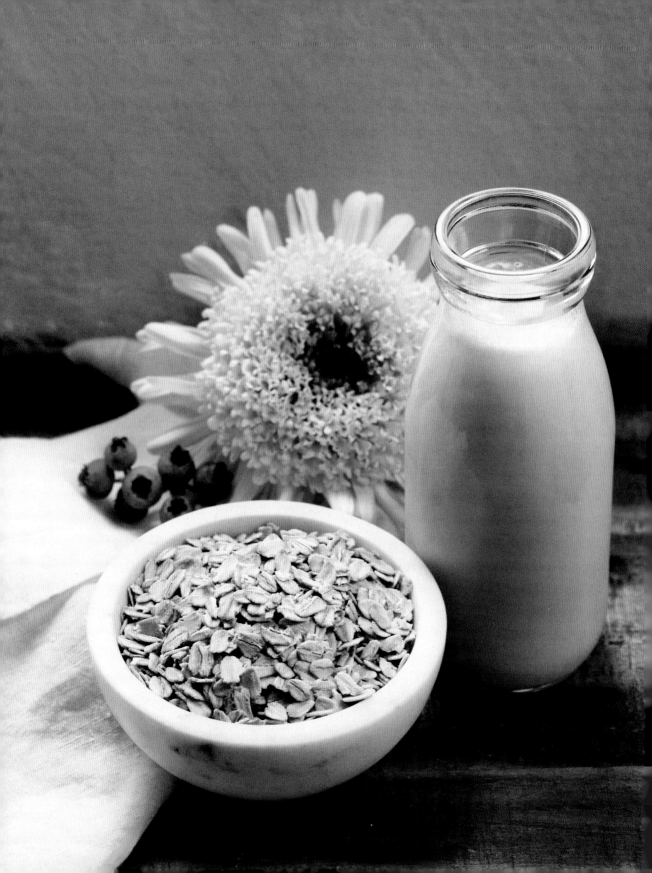

OAT MILK

oats

When breastfeeding, a lot of moms choose or have been advised to avoid dairy because of their own sensitivities or Baby's. Especially if you are used to eating dairy as part of your usual diet, going dairy-free on top of all the changes that already come with a new baby can be overwhelming. We often opt for non-dairy milks ourselves, but they can leave us craving the rich texture of cow's milk. Oat milk does such a fantastic job mimicking that creaminess, you'll even love it with your cereal. It also blends exceptionally well with coffee, tea, smoothies, and the like. Make a big batch and keep it in a mason jar in your fridge.

SERVES 2

1 cup organic old-fashioned rolled oats

1. Place the oats and 2 cups of water in a blender and blend for 30 seconds.

2. Strain, using a cheesecloth placed over a sieve, then strain again to remove all particles. Store in the refrigerator in an airtight container, such as a mason jar, for up to a week. Serve chilled.

VARIATION:

Chocolate Oat Milk

Along with the oats and water, add 1 tablespoon of pure maple syrup, 3 teaspoons of unsweetened cocoa powder, and ½ teaspoon of pure vanilla extract before blending.

Tip: Make a mocha café au lait by adding this variation to your morning coffee.

FENNEL-INFUSED COLD BREW

fennel seeds

A lot of debate and confusion surrounds caffeine and milk production. There is no evidence to support that caffeine intake directly decreases milk supply. However, drinking too much caffeine (more than 750 mg daily) can lead to an overstimulated baby who may not nurse well, and it can certainly be dehydrating for Mom. So, as with everything, we suggest drinking caffeine in moderation. Pediatricians suggest starting with 200 mg a day, and as Baby grows, he or she can better metabolize any caffeine in your diet. For those coffee-lovers, here is an absolutely delicious concoction that has about 75 mg of caffeine, with the added boost of fennel.

FENNEL SYRUP:

MAKES ABOUT ½ CUP SYRUP

1 cup water

2 tablespoons fennel seeds

⅓ cup coconut sugar

INFUSED COLD BREW:

SERVES 1

⅓ cup cold brew concentrate

⅔ cup whole milk or non-dairy milk of choice

2 teaspoons fennel syrup

1. Prepare the fennel syrup: Place the water and the fennel seeds and sugar in a small saucepan over medium-high heat. Let the mixture come to a boil and then lower the heat to medium.

2. Allow the mixture to simmer, stirring occasionally, for 8 to 10 minutes, or until the liquid is reduced by half and has become a dark and glossy syrup.

3. Pour the syrup through a fine-mesh strainer into a glass to remove the fennel seeds.

4. When you're ready to enjoy, combine the cold brew concentrate, milk, and 2 teaspoons of the fennel syrup, top the glass with ice, and stir. Enjoy immediately.

Note: Leftover fennel syrup will stay fresh in the refrigerator in an airtight container for up to 2 weeks.

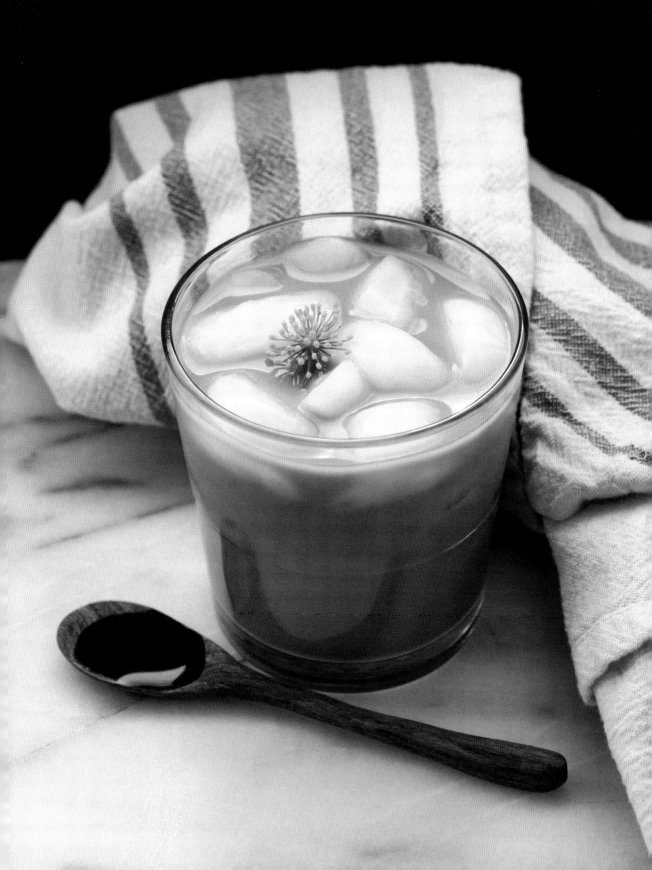

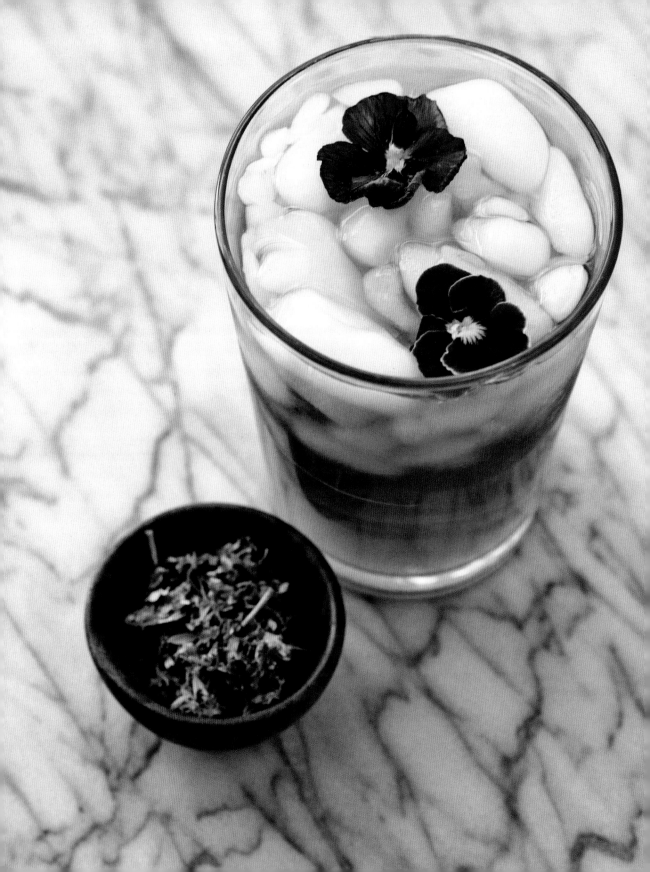

DIY LACTATION ICED TEA

fennel, raspberry leaves, nettle leaves

Sitting down to leisurely sip a warm beverage is not always in the cards for a busy new mom. Having a lactation tea that you can take on the go, in the car, and on a power walk can save the day. Not to mention, it is challenging to fit in three or four cups of hot tea in a day, but no problem at all to down that much iced tea in a single nursing session. Enjoying lactation tea cold means you'll drink it more often and you'll drink more of it, greatly increasing the chances you'll reap its milk-boosting benefits. Drink as is in place of water or play with it by sweetening with fresh fruit juice or honey or infusing it with slices of citrus.

MAKES 6 SERVINGS

2 fennel tea bags

2 raspberry leaf tea bags

2 nettle leaf tea bags

1. Bring 6 cups of water to a boil in a large pot.

2. Place the tea bags in a 2-quart mason jar or tempered glass pitcher. Pour the hot water over the tea bags and allow to steep for 10 minutes.

3. Remove and discard the tea bags.

4. Allow the tea to come to room temperature before covering with a lid or plastic wrap. Store in the refrigerator for up to a week. Enjoy over ice.

APRICOT GINGER SODA

apricots, ginger

We can't think of a drink more energizing than a sparkling fresh ginger soda. With just the right amount of bite from the grated ginger, and naturally sweetened with fresh apricot, this soda is the ideal accompaniment to a picnic lunch on a sunny afternoon. It is also ideal for easing indigestion, nausea, and fighting colds and flus, which can really do a number on your milk supply. Make the syrup in advance and store in the fridge, so you can whip up a tall, cold glass of this tonic anytime the mood strikes.

APRICOT GINGER SYRUP:

MAKES ABOUT ½ CUP SYRUP

4 fresh apricots, pitted and chopped

1 teaspoon grated fresh ginger

1 tablespoon coconut sugar

TO SERVE:

SERVES 1

1 to 2 tablespoons apricot ginger syrup

12 ounces soda water

1. Prepare the syrup: In a small saucepan, combine ½ cup of water with all the syrup ingredients and place over medium heat. Bring to a low boil and then simmer for 8 to 10 minutes, or until the apricots break down.

2. Remove from the heat and then smash the apricots with a wooden spoon or potato masher.

3. Strain the apricot ginger mixture through cheesecloth into a small mason jar, making sure to squeeze out all the liquid.

4. To serve, add 1 to 2 tablespoons of apricot ginger syrup to a 12-ounce glass of soda water. Top with ice and serve immediately. Store the remaining syrup in the refrigerator in an airtight container for up to 1 week.

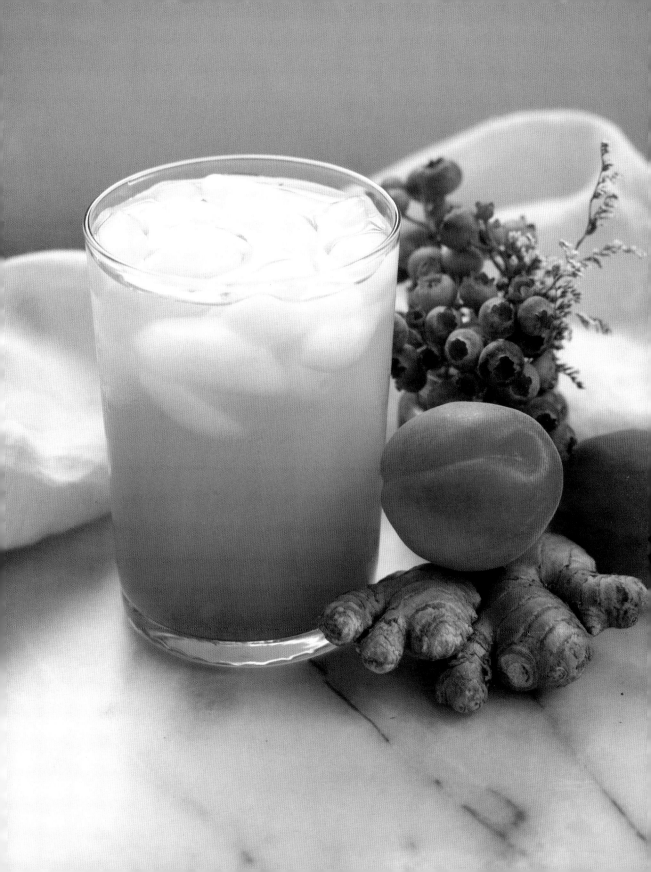

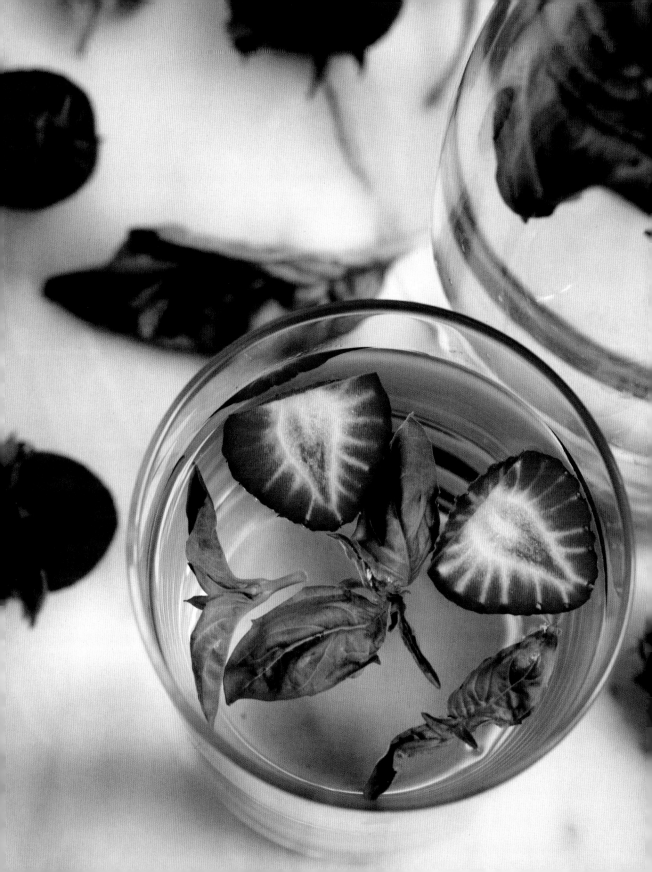

STRAWBERRY BASIL INFUSED WATER

basil

It seems like the moment we sit down to nurse, breastfeeding thirst kicks into high gear. Our mouth is parched and we can suddenly jug a gallon of water in one sitting. That's why it's important to always keep a hydrating beverage on hand at all times. Since many of us would like to avoid excess sugars in our drinks, infused waters help to keep fun flavors without the excess sugar.

MAKES 6 SERVINGS

4 to 6 fresh basil leaves

4 strawberries, hulled and sliced in half

6 cups filtered water

1. Gently pinch the basil leaves to help release their flavor. Place the basil along with the sliced strawberries in a wide-mouth 2-quart glass jar or pitcher.

2. Top up with the filtered water and allow to infuse in the refrigerator overnight. Enjoy straight or over ice.

Note: If you want to keep the infusion going, remove the strawberries and refresh with new ones every 2 days, with added water. Replace the basil after 3 days.

WATERMELON CHIA COOLER

chia seeds

If you are a fan of boba tea with tapioca, you're going to love this watermelon chia cooler. When chia seeds are soaked, they also turn into little balls of chewiness, adding a pleasing texture to your drink, and a ton of fiber as well. While tapioca offers little to no nutritional value, chia seeds are jam-packed with healthy fats and protein. Since watermelon is over 90 percent water, this drink will quench your breastfeeding thirst and ward off hunger at the same time.

SERVES 2

¼ cup chia seeds

3 cups fresh watermelon chunks

1½ teaspoons freshly squeezed lime juice

1½ teaspoons honey

1. In a small bowl, combine chia seeds with 1 cup of water and stir together. Set in the fridge to begin the gelling process. In about 30 minutes or so, whisk thoroughly until you've broken up any chunks and the seeds are well distributed in the water. Put back in the fridge and let sit for 2 to 3 hours or overnight.

2. When you're ready to make the cooler, place the watermelon, lime juice, and honey in a blender and blend until liquefied.

3. Pour the watermelon juice through a fine sieve and catch the juice in a bowl. Swirl watermelon mixture around the sieve to get as much juice as possible to drip through, but leave any watermelon pulp behind in the sieve.

4. Transfer the watermelon juice from the bowl to two glasses or jars. Add ½ cup of the soaked chia seeds to each glass. Whisk again to distribute the seeds throughout the juice. Enjoy cold. The cooler will stay fresh in a lidded mason jar in the refrigerator for 2 to 3 days.

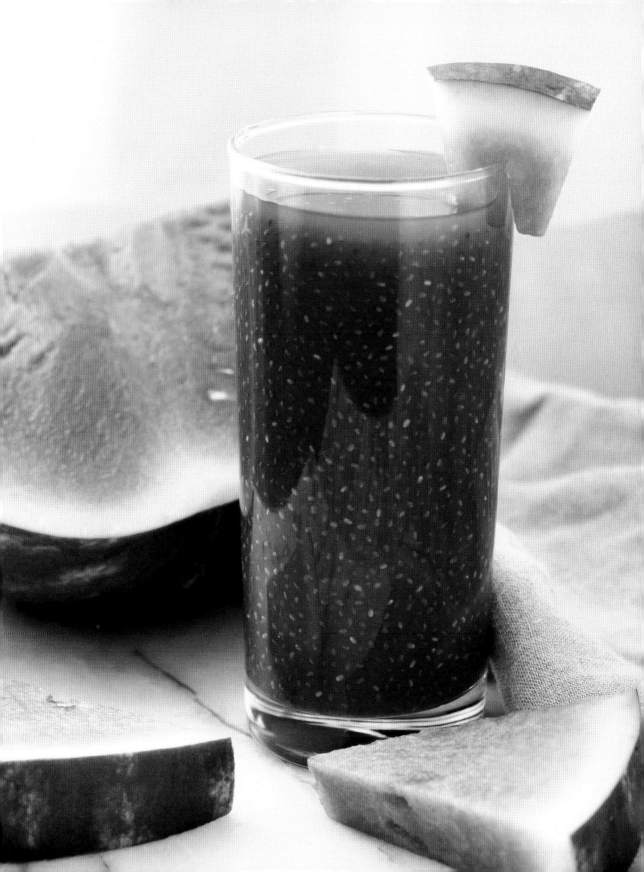

RESOURCES

RECOMMENDED READING

Latch: A Handbook for Breastfeeding with Confidence at Every Stage by Robin Kaplan (Berkeley: Rockridge Press, 2018)

The Nursing Mother's Companion by Kathleen Huggins (Cambridge: Harvard Common Press, 2017)

The Womanly Art of Breastfeeding by Diane Wiessinger, Diana West, and Teresa Pitman (New York: Ballantine Books, 2010)

Work. Pump. Repeat.: The New Mom's Survival Guide to Breastfeeding and Going Back to Work by Jessica Shortall (New York: Harry N. Abrams, 2015)

FIND SUPPORT NEAR YOU

International Lactation Consultant Association
https://www.ilca.org/why-ibclc/falc

La Leche League International
https://www.llli.org/get-help/

ACKNOWLEDGMENTS

We'd like to thank our customers and community of mamas who have rallied around us, our food, and our mission. Without you, there would be no Oat Mama. We'd also like to extend our thanks to our literary agent, editors, and publisher for bringing this book to life. We are thankful for Crissi and Nina of Milk and Honey for lending their expertise and to Mary Salas of @honeywild blog for sharing her beautiful breastfeeding images. Finally our hearts are full of love and gratitude for our partners, Alan and Mark, and for our five sweet boys. You make life worth living.

INDEX

Note: Page references in *italics* indicate photographs.

ABOUT THE AUTHORS

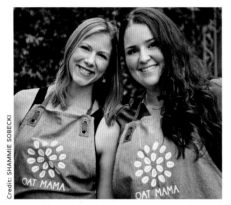

Credit: SHAMMIE SOBECKI

Eliza and Kristy met at a park while they were both pregnant with their second babies. They became fast friends, bonding over two-year-old tantrums, pregnancy woes, and their love of delicious food, of course. After baby number two came along, and they both began nursing again, they became fascinated with traditional lactogenic whole foods and herbs. They couldn't find much inspiration out there, so they decided to start their own lactation foods company Oat Mama. In just three short years, Oat Mama has grown into a million-dollar brand, featuring both lactation granola bars and teas, with a vibrant, ever-growing community of tens of thousands of breastfeeding moms looking for lactation food inspiration.